# Cancer Chemotherapy

# Cancer Chemotherapy

**Alan C. Sartorelli,** EDITOR

*Yale University*

A symposium sponsored by the
Division of Medicinal Chemistry
at the 169th Meeting of the
American Chemical Society,
Philadelphia, Pa.,
April 7, 1975.

ACS SYMPOSIUM SERIES / **30**

AMERICAN CHEMICAL SOCIETY
WASHINGTON, D. C.        1976

SEP

C HEM

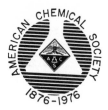

ad
12/7/76

Library of Congress CIP Data

Cancer chemotherapy

 (ACS symposium series; 30 ISSN 0097-6156)

 Includes biographical references and index.
 1. Cancer—chemotherapy.
 I. Sartorelli, Alan Clayton, 1931-        II. Series:
American Chemical Society. ACS symposium series; 30.
 DNLM: 1. Antineoplastic agents—Therapeutic use—
Congresses. 2. Neoplasms—Drug therapy—Congresses.

QZ267              C215                    1975
RC271.C5C292       616.9'94'061            76-24825
ISBN 0-8412-0336-9       ACSMC8 30 1-126 (1976)

# ACS Symposium Series

## Robert F. Gould, *Editor*

# FOREWORD

The ACS SYMPOSIUM SERIES was founded in 1974 to provide a medium for publishing symposia quickly in book form. The format of the SERIES parallels that of the continuing ADVANCES IN CHEMISTRY SERIES except that in order to save time the papers are not typeset but are reproduced as they are submitted by the authors in camera-ready form. As a further means of saving time, the papers are not edited or reviewed except by the symposium chairman, who becomes editor of the book. Papers published in the ACS SYMPOSIUM SERIES are original contributions not published elsewhere in whole or major part and include reports of research as well as reviews since symposia may embrace both types of presentation.

# CONTENTS

# PREFACE

Clinical results of the past decade have demonstrated that the use of chemical agents, largely in various combinations, in the treatment of disseminated cancer of man has resulted in a significant cure rate of various neoplasms, particularly the rapidly proliferating cancers of childhood. Thus, diseases such as acute lymphocytic leukemia, Ewing's sarcoma, Hodgkin's disease, choriocarcinoma, embryonal rhabdomyosarcoma, Burkitt's lymphoma, Wilms' tumor, and testicular carcinoma have responded dramatically to chemotherapy. Progress has been less spectacular with the more slowly growing neoplasms, e.g., carcinoma of the breast, lung, and colon, which comprise the major socioeconomic problems created by cancer.

To combat these forms of malignancy, considerable hope is placed upon the use of mixed modality therapy; the conceptual approach of such therapy is to lessen the neoplastic cell burden of the host by use of surgery and/or irradiation followed by chemotherapy designed to attack metastatic neoplastic cells. Although gains are to be expected from such therapeutic onslaughts, it seems reasonable to predict that addition of new agents to our therapeutic armamentarium will be of value. Thus, agents with biochemical mechanisms of action different from those currently used in the clinic are to be sought, as well as molecular modifications of existing agents designed to increase the therapeutic differential between the cancer and the host. In addition, the medicinal chemist may be required to design drugs with new actions. For example, potent antiviral agents may ultimately be necessary as part of the treatment of diseases such as acute leukemia. Therapeutic approaches leading to extensive prolongation of survival or cure, which rely on the extensive use of irradiation, alkylating agents, and/or other mutagens will be expected to induce new cancers; therefore, effort will necessarily be required to develop drugs capable of preventing carcinogenesis. Finally, noncytotoxic therapies must be devised; here, concepts such as differentiation therapy designed to convert neoplastic cells to less or noncancerous cells should be considered.

The proceedings of this symposium represent a sampling of a segment of the current approaches to the development of new and more efficacious antitumor drugs. The first chapter represents a class of agents, $\alpha$-(N)-heterocyclic carboxaldehyde thiosemicarbazones, which in theory should provide a useful derivative for the treatment of cancer, since the molecular target for these agents, the enzyme ribonucleoside diphosphate reductase, is of great importance to the synthesis of DNA and cell replication.

Adriamycin, perhaps the most exciting drug to appear in cancer therapy recently, has a wide spectrum of anticancer activity, particularly affecting several solid tumors. The rate-limiting cardiac toxicity of this material presents a challenge to medicinal chemistry, for it seems quite reasonable to assume that the molecular determinants of this toxicity to the heart are different than those responsible for cytotoxicity to tumor tissue. Thus, structural modification to minimize or eliminate cardiac toxicity should enhance considerably its clinical usefulness. For this reason, two chapters are included on this important antibiotic.

The alkylating agents represent an old class of highly active agents in which many derivatives have been synthesized and tested. Should additional compounds with this type of reactivity be designed and synthesized? The answer is clearly affirmative if unique carriers of the alkylating moiety, which direct alkylating potential largely to different cellular targets, are employed, or if other concepts are used to enhance anticancer specificity. The next chapter addresses itself to this latter possibility, attempting in its consideration of design principle, to take advantage of the anticipated higher reducing potential of hypoxic cells of solid tumors.

The last chapter represents an important discovery of recent years, the nitrosoureas, a class of agents which possesses both alkylating and carbamoylating activity. These materials represent a particular challenge in drug design, since a large number of these compounds are clinically active, and selection of additional members of this class for trial in man has become particularly difficult. Thus, as an aid to such a selection, it is extremely important to understand the relative importance of both alkylating and carbamoylating activities to anticancer potency, as well as to formulate an understanding of the intracellular molecular target(s) of these materials and the structural features which dictate tissue specificity.

It is to be expected that the tools of medicinal chemistry, particularly when guided by those of biochemistry and pharmacology, will provide new and better anticancer agents, and that the use of these materials with other drugs and treatment modalities will ultimately allow an expansion of the cure rate of various kinds of malignancy.

November 5, 1975                                   ALAN C. SARTORELLI

# Development of α-(N)-Heterocyclic Carboxaldehyde Thiosemicarbazones with Clinical Potential as Antineoplastic Agents

ALAN C. SARTORELLI and KRISHNA C. AGRAWAL

Department of Pharmacology and Section of Developmental Therapeutics, Division of Oncology, Yale University School of Medicine, New Haven, Conn. 06510

The initial report of the antineoplastic activity of an α-(N)-heterocyclic carboxaldehyde thiosemicarbazone was made in 1956 by Brockman and his associates (1) who reported that 2-formylpyridine thiosemicarbazone (PT) produced an increase in the life span of mice bearing the L1210 leukemia; the further development of this compound as a potential cancer chemotherapeutic agent was curtailed, however, because of its relatively low therapeutic index. Several years later, French and Blanz (2,3) described the synthesis of 1-formylisoquinoline thiosemicarbazone (IQ-1) and a variety of other α-(N)-heterocyclic carboxaldehyde thiosemicarbazones. These investigations demonstrated that several heterocyclic ring systems, including pyridine, isoquinoline, quinazoline, phthalazine, pyrazine, pyridazine, and purine possessed significant antineoplastic activity when the carbonyl attachment of the side chain was located at a position α to the ring nitrogen atom; attachment of the side chain β or γ to the heterocyclic N atom resulted in inactive antitumor agents.

Members of this class have shown anticancer activity against a wide spectrum of transplanted rodent neoplasms, including Sarcoma 180, Ehrlich carcinoma, Leukemia L1210, Lewis lung carcinoma, Hepatoma 129, Hepatoma 134, Adenocarcinoma 755, and B16 melanoma. In addition, spontaneous lymphomas of dogs have shown susceptibility to α-(N)-heterocyclic carboxaldehyde thiosemicarbazones. Such broad spectrum activity denotes great clinical potential and suggests that a drug of this class may well have utility in cancer therapy.

Extensive modification of the formyl thiosemicarbazone side chain of IQ-1 was carried out by Agrawal and Sartorelli (4) to ascertain the importance of this part of the molecule for anticancer activity. A variety of the substitutions and alterations of the various positions of the side chain that were made are shown in Figure 1; these changes uniformly led to complete loss or marked decrease in tumor-inhibitory potency. In addition, replacement of the heterocyclic ring N with C also resulted in a biologically inactive compound. These findings indicated the

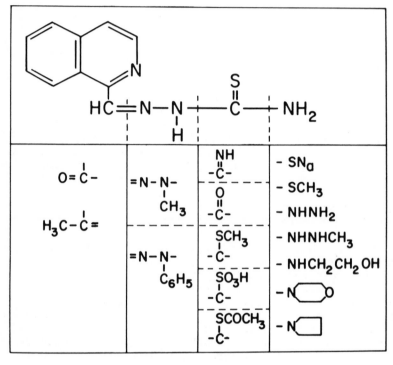

*Figure 1. Some modifications of the side chain of 1-formylisoquinoline thiosemicarbazone*

essentiality of this portion of the molecule and supported the
initial suggestion of French and Blanz (3) that a conjugate
N*-N*-S* tridentate ligand system was a requisite for tumor inhibitory activity.

   Extensive substitution of the isoquinoline and pyridine ring
systems of ∝-(N)-heterocyclic carboxaldehyde thiosemicarbazones
has been carried out by our laboratory (5-10) and by Blanz et al.
(11,12). A detailed summary of the effects of some of these substituents on antineoplastic efficacy has been reported (13,14).
Unfortunately, these investigations have not allowed detailed
predictions to be made concerning the importance of these modifications to the activity of this class of agents against neoplastic cells.

   The ∝-(N)-heterocyclic carboxaldehyde thiosemicarbazones
are strong coordinating agents for a number of transition metals
including divalent iron, cobalt, nickel, copper, zinc, and man-
ganese (3). The crystal structure of bis(isoquinoline-1-carbox-
aldehyde thiosemicarbazanato)nickel (II) monohydrate has been determined (15), with the findings indicating that the nickel atom
is octahedrally coordinated by the two approximately planar tridentate IQ-1 ligands.

   A number of laboratories have studied the metal ion interactions of PT (16-18) and 5-hydroxy-2-formylpyridine thiosemicarbazone (5-HP) and its selenosemicarbazone, guanylhydrazone and
semicarbazone analogs (19). The stoichiometry for the interaction of PT with Fe(II) has been reported to be three molecules of
ligand (16,17) to one atom of metal, with the most stable complex
having a stability constant of log $\beta$ = 44.9. The exceptionally
strong affinity of ∝-(N)-heterocyclic carboxaldehyde thiosemicarbazones for iron was demonstrated in vivo by French et al.
(20) who reported that administration to mice of a dose of 100 mg
of 2-formylpyrazine thiosemicarbazone per kg resulted in the
urinary excretion of about 11 ug of iron in 24 hours, and by
DeConti et al. (21) and Krakoff et al. (22) who showed that
treatment of cancer patients with 5-HP led to the excretion of
significant amounts of iron (2 to 11 mg/24 hours) in the urine,
presumably in chelate form with 5-HP. A direct correlation between chelating abilities of ∝-(N)-heterocyclic carboxaldehyde
thiosemicarbazones and their antitumor activities has been shown
(19,23). The antitumor effects of transition metal chelates of
IQ-1 have also been reported; in these investigations, the iron
chelate of IQ-1 was found to be the most potent inhibitor of DNA
synthesis of several chelates tested (24).

Biochemical Mechanism of Action

   The ∝-(N)-heterocyclic carboxaldehyde thiosemicarbazones
constitute, as a class, the most potent known inhibitors of ribonucleoside diphosphate reductase, being 80- to 5000-times more
effective than the classical inhibitor of this enzyme, hydroxyurea

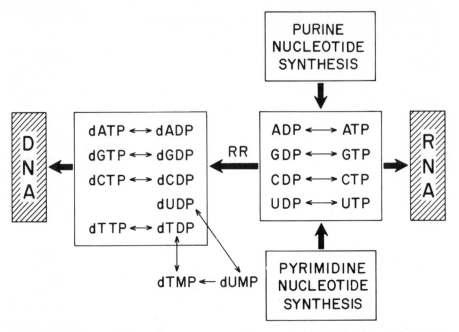

*Figure 2. Relationship of ribonucleoside diphosphate reductase (RR) to the synthesis of DNA*

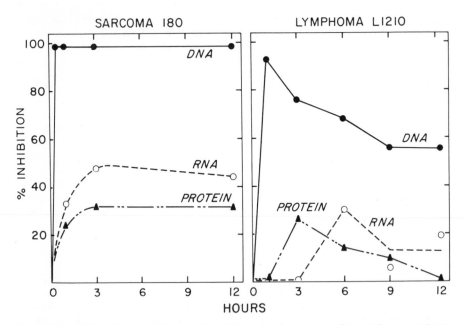

*Figure 3. Effect of 1-formylisoquinoline thiosemicarbazone on the syntheses of DNA, RNA, and protein of Sarcoma 180 and Leukemia L1210*

(25). The reductive conversion of ribonucleotides to deoxyribonucleotides by this enzyme is a particularly critical step in the
synthesis of DNA, since deoxyribonucleotides which are generated
through this enzymatic reduction are present in extremely low
levels in mammalian cells.  The central position of ribonucleotide reductase to the synthesis of DNA is illustrated in Figure
2. The relative importance of such a reaction to neoplastic cell
reproduction has been demonstrated by Elford et al. (26) in a
series of rat hepatomas of different growth rates.  A positive
correlation occurs in these tumors between growth rate and activity of ribonucleotide reductase; whereas, two other enzymes of
importance to DNA biosynthesis, thymidylate synthetase and thymidine kinase, did not demonstrate such a close degree of correlation with tumor growth.  Thus, it seems reasonable that a strong
inhibitor of ribonucleoside diphosphate reductase would be a useful weapon in the therapeutic armamentarium against cancer.

Blockade of ribonucleotide reductase by $\alpha$-(N)-heterocyclic
carboxaldehyde thiosemicarbazones results in inhibition of DNA
biosynthesis, which is the primary site of action of these agents
(27,28); therefore, these agents exert their action in the S
phase of the cell cycle (29,30).  Inhibition of the synthesis of
RNA and protein by $\alpha$-(N)-heterocyclic carboxaldehyde thiosemicarbazones can be demonstrated; however, these processes are considerably less sensitive than is the biosynthesis of DNA (27,28,
31-33).  The relative sensitivities of these biosynthetic
processes to IQ-1 in Sarcoma 180 and Leukemia L1210 ascites cells
is shown in Figure 3.  In Sarcoma 180, essentially complete inhibition of thymidine-H$^3$ incorporation into DNA was caused by a
single dose of 40 mg of IQ-1/kg; this degree of interference with
DNA biosynthesis continues for 12 hours and by 24 hours after the
drug, thymidine-H$^3$ incorporation has returned to control levels.
Depression of the incorporation of uridine-H$^3$ and leucine-C$^{14}$
into RNA and protein, respectively, by IQ-1 is delayed somewhat
and reaches a maximum degree of inhibition of 50 and 35%.  In the
L1210 leukemia, DNA biosynthesis appeared to be less sensitive to
IQ-1, with recovery occurring more rapidly; inhibition of
leucine-C$^{14}$ and uridine-H$^3$ incorporation into protein and RNA,
respectively, was delayed and relatively weak.

The localization of the site of inhibition of DNA biosynthesis at the level of ribonucleotide reductase is the result of a
series of investigations which demonstrated:  (a) that the conversion of thymidine-H$^3$ to deoxythymidine triphosphate (dTTP) in neoplastic cells was not decreased by $\alpha$-(N)-heterocyclic carboxaldehyde thiosemicarbazones, while the subsequent incorporation of
dTTP into DNA was markedly inhibited (31-33); (b) that incorporation of dTTP-H$^3$, in the presence of adequate concentrations of the
other three nonlabeled deoxyribonucleoside triphosphates, into
DNA of isolated tumor cell nuclei was not decreased by relatively
high concentrations of IQ-1 (28); and (c) that the incorporation
of cytidine-H$^3$ into cellular pyrimidine ribonucleotides was insen-

sitive to ∝-(N)-heterocyclic carboxaldehyde thiosemicarbazones;
whereas, the throughput of radioactivity from the ribonucleotide
pool into pyrimidine deoxyribonucleotides was strongly depressed
(31-33).

The kinetic mechanism of inhibition of ribonucleoside diphosphate reductase by ∝-(N)-heterocyclic carboxaldehyde thiosemicarbazones is not clear. The concentrations of the nucleoside
diphosphate substrate, the allosteric activator ATP, or magnesium
ion do not influence the inhibition of the enzyme produced by all
of the thiosemicarbazones tested to date. Interesting differences exist, however, between the ring hydroxylated and nonhydrox-
ylated ∝-(N)-heterocyclic carboxaldehyde thiosemicarbazones with
respect to the dithiols, used as model substrates in place of the
natural substrate thioredoxin, and to iron. IQ-1 and PT are
similar in action; both are partially competitive with the dithiol
substrate and both prevent any stimulation of reductase activity
by iron. It has been hypothesized (32,33) that inhibition by
these derivatives is the result of either coordination of iron in
the metal-charged enzyme by the inhibitor, or formation of an iron
chelate of IQ-1, which acts as the true inhibitor at or near the
site functionally occupied by thioredoxin.

Studies conducted on the inhibition of ribonucleotide reductase by the preformed iron chelate of IQ-1 [(Fe)IQ-1] at high and
low concentrations of $Fe^{++}$ (34) have shown that (Fe)IQ-1 inhibited enzymatic activity by 73% in the absence of added $Fe^{++}$, but
only 30% with $Fe^{++}$; whereas, IQ-1 decreased enzyme activity 65%
in the presence of thioredoxin and $Fe^{++}$, but only 40% without
thioredoxin and only 15% without $Fe^{++}$ (34). The findings imply
that Fe(II)IQ-1 is the active form of the inhibitor and stress
further the complexities of the mode of inhibition.

The hydroxylated derivatives, 5-HP and 3-hydroxy-2-formyl-
pyridine thiosemicarbazone, show a different pattern of inhibition (33). They appear "competitive" with iron and either non-
competitive or uncompetitive with the dithiol substrate; the im-
precise nature of the assay did not allow a choice between these
alternatives. The failure of the dithiol to reverse inhibition
of ribonucleoside diphosphate reductase by the hydroxylated derivatives implies that the interaction of these inhibitors with the
enzyme occurs at a site different from that involved in the
action of PT and IQ-1. The impure nature of this complex enzyme
system, however, makes it impossible to explain fully these differences and further advances will require the availability of a
highly purified enzyme.

Some of the structural features required for inhibition of
ribonucleoside diphosphate reductase have been determined (35).
These studies suggested that position 6 of PT and position 3 of
IQ-1 are equivalent with respect to orientation of the inhibitor
at the enzymatic binding site and that little or no tolerance
exists for modification at this position. In addition, substitution of the terminal amino group of the thiosemicarbazone side

chain decreased enzyme inhibition, supporting the presence of a low bulk tolerance zone in this position (36). The results also indicated that IQ-1, which can be visualized as a pyridine derivative with a benzene ring fused across the 3 and 4 positions, is about six-fold more potent as an inhibitor of the enzyme than is PT. Likewise, introduction of a $CH_3$ group on the pyridine ring of PT at either the 3, 4, or 5 positions resulted in derivatives that were better inhibitors of ribonucleoside diphosphate reductase activity than PT. These findings suggest the possible existence of a hydrophobic bonding zone adjacent to the inhibitor-binding site of the enzyme.

Although the primary biochemical lesion induced by the α-(N)-heterocyclic carboxaldehyde thiosemicarbazones appears to be at the level of the enzyme ribonucleoside diphosphate reductase, and studies of structure-activity relationships have indicated the requirement for inhibition of this enzyme for antineoplastic activity (14), recent studies from our laboratory have shown that IQ-1 interacts directly with Sarcoma 180 DNA and causes single strand breaks in DNA (37). This agrees with the findings of Karon and Benedict (30) who have reported that 5-HP caused chromatid breaks, primarily during the S-phase, in hamster fibroblasts. This second site of action, which may be the result of interference with reductase activity, appears to be of major significance to the cytotoxic mechanism of action of these agents, since it creates a lesion in the genome that is reinforced by blockade of ribonucleoside diphosphate reductase.

## Phase I Clinical Trials

It seems reasonable that a potent inhibitor of ribonucleoside diphosphate reductase would be an important addition to the chemotherapeutic arsenal for the treatment of rapidly growing cancers. In support of this, three different types of drugs with relatively weak inhibitory potency for ribonucleoside diphosphate reductase [i.e. hydroxyurea (38), guanazole (39), and 5-HP (33, 40,41)] have all demonstrated some, although clearly minimal, activity in man. 5-HP is the only member of this series that has been administered to man as part of a Phase I study (21,22). The selection of 5-HP for clinical trials was due to (a) its considerable activity against transplanted tumors (42,43) and a spontaneous dog lymphoma (44), and (b) its ease of parenteral administration as its sodium salt (45). The results of the two independent Phase I studies showed that transient decreases in blast counts occurred in 6 of 25 patients with leukemia, while no antitumor effects were observed in 18 patients with solid tumors. Administration of relatively large doses of drug was limited primarily by gastrointestinal toxicity; the clinical impression was that this toxicity was centrally mediated. In addition, the most aggressive drug regimens also produced myelosuppression, hemolysis, anemia, hypertension and hypotension. Thus, the impressive anti-

neoplastic activity of 5-HP in animal systems was not achieved
in man, although it must be stressed that in this instance, as in
all Phase I investigations, far advanced patients were employed.
The relative inactivity of 5-HP as an inhibitor of tumor growth
in man appeared to be the result of (a) its relatively low inhibitory potency for the target enzyme, ribonucleoside diphosphate
reductase, compared to the most potent member of this class, IQ-1,
being about 100-fold less effective, and (b) its short biological
half-life in man because of the rapid formation and elimination
of the o-glucuronide conjugate (21).
     The results presented in Table I show that the $t_{1/2}$ of 5-HP
in the blood of mice was 15 minutes, while the drug had a $t_{1/2}$ in
man of 2.5 to 10.5 minutes, depending upon the patient. Twenty
percent of a therapeutic dose of 5-HP was excreted in the urine
of the mouse in 24 hours; whereas, a therapeutic dose of 5-HP was
excreted 2- to 3.5-times faster in man. Approximately 75% of the
material found in the urine of man was in the form of an o-glucuronide.
     These investigations implied that the development of an effi-
cacious second generation α-(N)-heterocyclic carboxaldehyde thiosemicarbazone, which had (a) greater affinity for the target

Table I.  Comparative Blood Levels and Urinary Excretion of 5-
          Hydroxy-2-formylpyridine Thiosemicarbazone in Mice and
          Man

| Species | Blood Levels $t_{1/2}$ (min) | Urinary Excretion (% in 24 h) |
|---------|------------------------------|-------------------------------|
| Mice    | 15                           | 20                            |
| Man     | 2.5-10.5                     | 47-75                         |

enzyme, ribonucleoside diphosphate reductase, and (b) the
presence of a hydrophilic group other than a phenolic hydroxyl
function to provide for solubilization and formulation of these
extremely water-insoluble compounds, might lead to a useful antineoplastic agent.
     To synthesize agents that are not susceptible to enzymatic
inactivation by o-glucuronide formation, amino groups were added
to the heteroaromatic rings of both pyridine and isoquinoline
thiosemicarbazones. The amino function would permit water solubility as an acid salt. To enhance affinity for the target
enzyme, in the pyridine series, the hydrophobic phenyl ring was
introduced at various positions in 2-formylpyridine thiosemicarbazone in an effort to take advantage of the postulated hydrophobic interacting region between enzyme and inhibitor (46). The
effects of these derivatives on the survival time of mice bearing
Sarcoma 180 ascites cells and on the activity of ribonucleoside

diphosphate reductase from the Novikoff rat tumor are shown in
Table II. 2-Formyl-4-(m-amino)phenylpyridine thiosemicarbazone
possessed the optimum combination of structural features and was
the most active of the m-aminophenyl derivatives as an inhibitor
of both tumor-growth and ribonucleoside diphosphate reductase activity. The ortho- and para-substituted 4-aminophenylpyridine
thiosemicarbazones were also synthesized and tested for antineoplastic activity against Sarcoma 180 (47); both derivatives were

Table II.    Effect of Substituted 2-Formylpyridine Thiosemicarba-
             zones on the Survival Time of Mice Bearing Sarcoma 180
             Ascites Cells and on the Activity of Ribonucleoside
             Diphosphate Reductase from the Novikoff Rat Tumor

| Compound | Tumor-inhibitory activity | | Enzyme-inhibitory activity |
|---|---|---|---|
| | Maximum effective daily dosage (mg/kg)* | Av. survival time (days) | 50% inhibitory concentration (uM) |
| None | -- | 13.7 | -- |
| 2-Formylpyridine thiosemicarbazone (PT) | 2.5 | 16.1 | 0.40 |
| 3-(m-Aminophenyl) PT | 5 | 18.4 | 3.3 |
| 4-(m-Aminophenyl) PT | 40 | 32.5 | 0.11 |
| 5-(m-Aminophenyl) PT | 20 | 21.5 | 0.74 |
| 6-(m-Aminophenyl) PT | 20 | 13.6 | 55 |

*Administered once daily for 6 consecutive days beginning 24
hr after tumor implantation; dose levels were administered in
a range of 5-60 mg/kg for each compound.

essentially devoid of antitumor activity. The inactivity of the
ortho- and para-substituted amino derivatives conceivably is due
to mesomeric stabilization of cationic species which tend to
hinder the coordination of metals by the pair of free electrons
on the ring nitrogen (47).

      Molecular models of 3-, 4-, and 5-(m-aminophenyl)pyridine
thiosemicarbazone have been constructed in an effort to visual-
ize the critical portions of the inhibitor molecule for enzymatic
interaction; these structures are shown in Figure 4. The most
potent of these derivatives as an inhibitor of ribonucleotide reductase and of tumor growth, the 4-substituted molecule, is shown
in Panel B; the benzenoid ring constitutes the area of hypothetical interaction between enzyme and inhibitor. Panel A shows the
structure of 3-(m-aminophenyl)pyridine thiosemicarbazone; the
relatively poor inhibitory activity of this compound conceivably
results from the projection of the hydrophilic amino group into
the area of hydrophobic interaction. The intermediate potency of

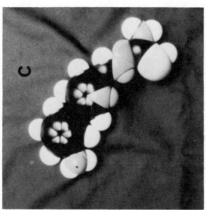

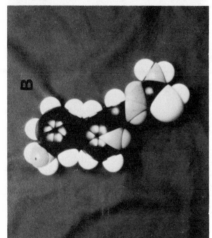

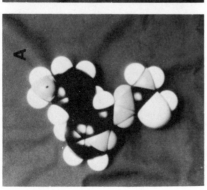

*Figure 4. Molecular models of 3-, 4-, and 5-(m-aminophenyl)pyridine thiosemicarbazone. A. 3-(m-aminophenyl)pyridine thiosemicarbazone; B. 4-(m-aminophenyl)pyridine thiosemicarbazone; C. 5-(m-aminophenyl)pyridine thiosemicarbazone*

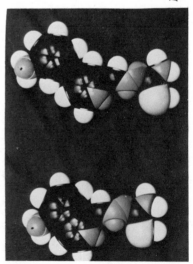

*Figure 5. Molecular models of 5-amino-1-formylisoquinoline thiosemicarbazone (left) and 4-(m-aminophenyl)pyridine thiosemicarbazone (right)*

the 5-aminophenyl substituted compound, Panel C, is possibly due
to the lack of significant contribution of the benzenoid nucleus
to the hydrophobic bonding between enzyme and inhibitor.

The 5-amino derivative of IQ-1 (5) also appeared to be a possible candidate as a second generation α-(N)-heterocyclic carboxaldehyde thiosemicarbazone with clinical potential in cancer
chemotherapy. The molecular models shown in Figure 5 demonstrate
the structural similarities between 5-amino IQ-1 and 4-(m-aminophenyl)pyridine thiosemicarbazone. 5-Amino IQ-1 required only
0.03 uM for 50% inhibition of the activity of ribonucleoside diphosphate reductase from the Novikoff hepatoma (48), making this
agent equal to IQ-1 itself as the most potent known inhibitor of
this enzyme. 5-Amino IQ-1 has, however, significant advantage
over IQ-1 in that it can be rendered soluble as an acidic salt.
The potent antineoplastic activity of 5-amino IQ-1 against Sarcoma
180 is shown in Table III.

Table III.   Effect of 5-Aminoisoquinoline-1-carboxaldehyde
             Thiosemicarbazone On the Survival Time of Mice
             Bearing Sarcoma 180 Ascites Cells

| Daily dose (mg/kg)* | Av. Δ wt. (%) | Av. survival time (days) | 50-Day survivors/total |
|---|---|---|---|
| 0 | +19.8 | 12.4 | 0/20 |
| 5 | + 3.1 | 27.0 | 0/5 |
| 10 | - 1.8 | 24.0 | 0/5 |
| 20 | - 7.8 | 27.4 | 0/5 |
| 40 | - 8.5 | 37.3 | 3/10 |

*Tumor-bearing mice were treated once daily with the indicated
 dose for 6 consecutive days beginning 24 hours after the
 transplantation of about 6 x $10^6$ tumor cells.

Similar studies have demonstrated that Leukemia L1210, Leukemia
P388, Hepatoma 129, Ehrlich carcinoma and B16 Melanoma are also
susceptible to the tumor-inhibitory properties of 5-amino IQ-1.

Since acetylation, a common enzymatic reaction, of the amino
function of 5-amino IQ-1 results in loss of tumor-inhibitory potency, a methyl group was introduced at the 4-position of the
isoquinoline ring to create steric hinderance to acetylating enzymes, as well as to other possible enzymatic alterations (49).
Incubation of 5-amino-1-methylisoquinoline and 5-amino-1,4-dimeth-
ylisoquinoline with acetyl coenzyme A and rat liver homogenate
resulted in about 20-fold higher acetylation of 5-amino-1-
methylisoquinoline. A similar experiment conducted with 5-amino
IQ-1 and 4-methyl-5-amino IQ-1 was complicated by acetylation
of the terminal thioamide group. 4-Methyl-5-amino IQ-1 was

essentially equal to 5-amino IQ-1 as an antineoplastic agent in
a number of transplanted rodent tumor systems and as an inhibitor
of ribonucleoside diphosphate reductase.  These findings, as well
as the protection afforded the ring-substituted amino function by
the relatively bulky methyl group, makes 4-methyl-5-amino IQ-1
a prime candidate as the second generation drug of this class for
clinical trial.

## Literature Cited

1.  Brockman, R. W., Thomson, J. R., Bell, M. J., and Skipper,
    H. E., Cancer Res., (1956) 16, 167-170.
2.  French, F. A., and Blanz, E. J., Jr., Cancer Res., (1965)
    25, 1454-1458.
3.  French, F. A., and Blanz, E. J., Jr., J. Med. Chem., (1966)
    9, 585-589.
4.  Agrawal, K. C., and Sartorelli, A. C., J. Med. Chem., (1969)
    12, 771-774.
5.  Agrawal, K. C., Booth, B. A., and Sartorelli, A. C., J.
    Med. Chem., (1968) 11, 700-703.
6.  Agrawal, K. C., Cushley, R. J., McMurray, W. J., and
    Sartorelli, A. C., J. Med. Chem., (1970) 13, 431-434.
7.  Agrawal, K. C., Cushley, R. J., Lipsky, S. R., Wheaton, J.
    R., and Sartorelli, A. C., J. Med. Chem., (1972) 15, 192-
    195.
8.  Lin, A. J., Agrawal, K. C., and Sartorelli, A. C., J. Med.
    Chem., (1972) 15, 615-618.
9.  Agrawal, K. C., Booth, B. A., Moore, E. C., and Sartorelli,
    A. C., J. Med. Chem., (1972) 15, 1154-1158.
10. Agrawal, K. C., Booth, B. A., and Sartorelli, A. C., J. Med.
    Chem., (1973) 16, 715-717.
11. French, F. A., Blanz, E. J., Jr., DoAmaral, J. R., and
    French, D. A., J. Med. Chem., (1970) 13, 1117-1124.
12. Blanz, E. J., Jr., French, F. A., DoAmaral, J. R., and
    French, D. A., J. Med. Chem., (1970) 13, 1124-1130.
13. French, F. A., and Blanz, E. J., Jr., Cancer Chemother.
    Rep., (1971) 2, 199-235.
14. Agrawal, K. C., and Sartorelli, A. C., in, Sartorelli, A.
    C., and Johns, D. G., Handbook of Experimental Pharmacology,
    38 (Part II), 791-807, Springer-Verlag, Berlin (1975).
15. Mathew, M., and Palenik, G. J., J. Am. Chem. Soc., (1969)
    91, 6310-6314.
16. Cano, J. M., Benito, D. P., and Pino, E., Quimica, (1971)
    67, 299-307.
17. Leggett, D. J., and McBryde, W. A. E., Talanta, (1975) 22,
    in press.
18. Anthroline, W., and Petering, D. H., Proc. Am. Assoc. Cancer
    Res., (1974) 15, 16.
19. Agrawal, K. C., Booth, B. A., Michaud, R. L., Moore, E. C.,
    and Sartorelli, A. C., Biochem. Pharmacol., (1974) 23, 2421-

2429.

20. French, F. A., Lewis, A. E., Sheena, A. H., and Blanz, E. J., Jr., Fed. Proc., (1965) 24, 402.
21. DeConti, R. C., Toftness, B. R., Agrawal, K. C., Tomchick, R., Mead, J. A. R., Bertino, J. R., Sartorelli, A. C., and Creasey, W. A., Cancer Res., (1972) 32, 1455-1462.
22. Krakoff, I. H., Etcubanas, E., Tan, C., Mayer, K., Bethune, V., and Burchenal, J. H., Cancer Chemoth. Rep., (1974) 58, 207-212.
23. Michaud, R. L., and Sartorelli, A. C., Abstracts of Papers, 155th Amer. Chem. Soc. National Meeting, No. NO54, San Francisco, April (1968).
24. Agrawal, K. C., Booth, B. A., Moore, E. C., and Sartorelli, A. C., Proc. Am. Assoc. Cancer Res., (1974) 15, 73.
25. Sartorelli, A. C., Cancer Res., (1969) 29, 2292-2299.
26. Elford, H. L., Freeze, M., Passamani, E., and Morris, H. P., J. Biol. Chem., (1970) 245, 5228-5233.
27. Sartorelli, A. C., Biochem. Biophys. Res. Communs., (1967) 27, 26-32.
28. Sartorelli, A. C., Hilton, J., Booth, B. A., Agrawal, K. C., Donnelly, T. E., Jr., and Moore, E. C., Adv. Biol. Skin, (1972) 12, 271-285.
29. Bhuyan, B. K., Scheidt, L. G., Fraser, T. J., Cancer Res., (1972) 32, 398-407.
30. Karon, M., and Benedict, W. F., Science, (1972) 178, 62.
31. Booth, B. A., Moore, E. C., and Sartorelli, A. C., Cancer Res., (1971) 31, 228-234.
32. Moore, E. C., Zedeck, M. S., Agrawal, K. C., and Sartorelli, A. C., Biochem., (1970) 9, 4492-4498.
33. Moore, E. C., Booth, B. A., and Sartorelli, A. C., Cancer Res., (1971) 31, 235-238.
34. Moore, E. C., Agrawal, K. C., and Sartorelli, A. C., Proc. Am. Assoc. Cancer Res., (1975) 16, 160.
35. Sartorelli, A. C., Agrawal, K. C., and Moore, E. C., Biochem. Pharmacol., (1971) 20, 3119-3123.
36. Agrawal, K. C., Lee, M. H., Booth, B. A., Moore, E. C., and Sartorelli, A. C., J. Med. Chem., (1974) 17, 934-938.
37. Tsiftsoglou, A. S., Hwang, K. M., Agrawal, K. C., and Sartorelli, A. C., Biochem. Pharmacol., (1975) in press.
38. Krakoff, I. H., in Sartorelli, A. C., and Johns, D. G., Handbook of Experimental Pharmacology, 38 (Part II), 789-792, Springer-Verlag, Berlin (1975).
39. Brockman, R. W., Shaddix, S., Laster, W. R., Jr., and Schabel, F. M., Jr., Cancer Res., (1970) 30, 2358-2368.
40. Sartorelli, A. C., Booth, B. A., and Moore, E. C., Proc. Am. Assoc. Cancer Res., (1969) 10, 76.
41. Brockman, R. W., Sidwell, R. W., Arnett, G., and Shaddix, S., Proc. Soc. Exptl. Biol. Med., (1970) 133, 609-614.
42. French, F. A., and Blanz, E. J., Jr., Gann, (1967) 2, 51-57.

43. Blanz, E. J., Jr., and French, F. A., Cancer Res., (1968)
    28, 2419-2422.
44. Creasey, W. A., Agrawal, K. C., Capizzi, R. L., Stinson,
    K. K., and Sartorelli, A. C., Cancer Res., (1972) 32, 565-
    572.
45. Agrawal, K. C., and Sartorelli, A. C., J. Pharm. Sci., (1968)
    57, 1948-1951.
46. Agrawal, K. C., Lin, A. J., Booth, B. A., Wheaton, J. R.,
    and Sartorelli, A. C., J. Med. Chem., (1974) 17, 631-635.
47. Agrawal, K. C., Booth, B. A., DeNuzzo, S. M., and Sartorelli,
    A. C., J. Med. Chem., (1975) 18, 368-371.
48. Mooney, P. D., Booth, B. A., Moore, E. C., Agrawal, K. C.,
    and Sartorelli, A. C., J. Med. Chem., (1974) 17, 1145-1150.
49. Agrawal, K. C., Mooney, P. D., Schenkman, J. B., Denk, H.,
    Moore, E. C., and Sartorelli, A. C., Pharmacologist, (1975)
    17, 201.

# Adriamycin

DAVID W. HENRY

Stanford Research Institute, Menlo Park, Calif. 94025

Introduction. Adriamycin (1, also called doxorubicin) is an anthracycline antibiotic and was first isolated in the late 1960s by Arcamone and colleagues in the Farmitalia research laboratories (1,2). It is produced by a mutant strain of Streptomyces peucetius, the microorganism that produces the closely related antibiotic daunomycin (2). Daunomycin (also known as rubidomycin, daunorubicin and rubomycin) was independently discovered in three laboratories several years earlier than adriamycin (3-5) and has

1  R = OH  adriamycin
2  R = H   daunomycin

achieved a significant place in the treatment of acute lymphocytic and myelogenous leukemias (6,7). Adriamycin is also an active antileukemic drug but is of much greater interest because of its activity against a broad spectrum of solid tumors (8-10). It is the objective of this paper to briefly summarize significant background data on the chemical, biochemical and clinical properties of adriamycin and daunomycin and subsequently to describe more fully the status of structure-activity studies stemming from the

parent antibiotics.  It is appropriate and necessary to include
considerable information on daunomycin because of the close
relationship between the chemical and biochemical properties of
the two antibiotics and because daunomycin has been available for
study longer than adriamycin.

The anthracycline antibiotics are produced by the strepo-
mycetes and are characterized by the presence of a tetrahydronaphthacene quinone moiety.  They bear several additional oxygen
functions in the aromatic and saturated portions of the aglycone
and variation in the number and position of these substituents
(usually hydroxyls) distinguish individual compounds.  Many members of this group are known, largely through the work of
Brockmann (11,12).  Significant cytotoxic activity is almost
always associated with basic glycosides of the parent nucleus,
rather than the aglycones themselves, and complete structural
information is often lacking for these sugar conjugates.  A
second group of anthracyclines with in vitro and/or in vivo cytotoxic character are given in Figure 1.  With the exception of
carminomycin, these compounds have been studied comparatively
little and they will not be further discussed in any detail.
Carminomycin (3) has received much attention in the USSR (13-21)
since first reported by Gauze et al. in 1973 and data on it will
be cited where pertinent.

Chemistry.  The structural assignment of adriamycin rests
heavily on a correlation with that of daunomycin (22).  Mild
acidic hydrolysis of adriamycin yields the aglycone, adriamycinone (8, Figure 2), and the amino sugar, daunosamine (10).
The ultraviolet and visible spectra of 8 were identical to those
of the parent and daunomycin, thus establishing the chromophore
structure.  Detailed spectral analyses of 8, 7-deoxy-adria-
mycinone (9), bisanhydroadriamycinone (11), and their acetylation
products further established the close relationship to daunomycin
and fixed the position of the additional hydroxyl group in the
acetyl side chain.

The structure of daunomycin was established in two stages.
The original chemical publications by Arcamone et al. (23,24)
described the hydrolysis to the aglycone, daunomycinone, and the
amino sugar, daunosamine.  The major structural features of
daunomycinone were determined by a combination of spectral analyses and chemical degradation, leaving the stereochemistry of the
tetrahydro ring and the locations of the methoxy and glycosidic
groups unspecified.  Several years later (25,26) the Italian
group completed the structural assignments of daunomycinone by a
further degradative sequence yielding 1,6,10,11-tetrahydroxy-
naphthacene-5,12-dione derivatives (e.g., 12) whose spectral
properties specified the correct hydroxylation pattern.  Simultaneously they succeeded in fixing the glycosidic link at the 7-
hydroxy by careful nmr analysis of daunomycin pentaacetate and
by catalytic reduction of daunomycin to 7-deoxydaunomycinone.

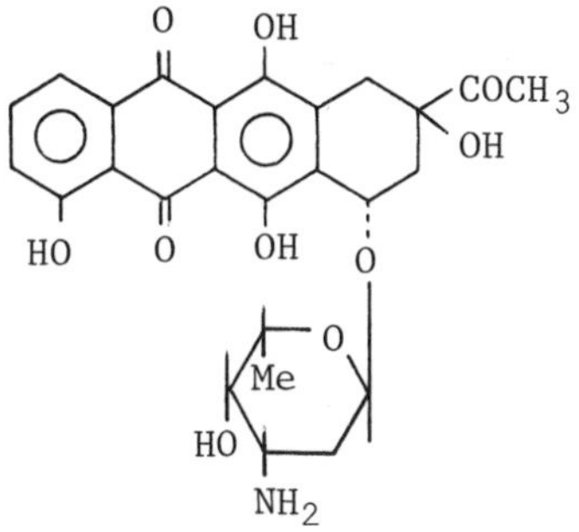

3 carminomycin

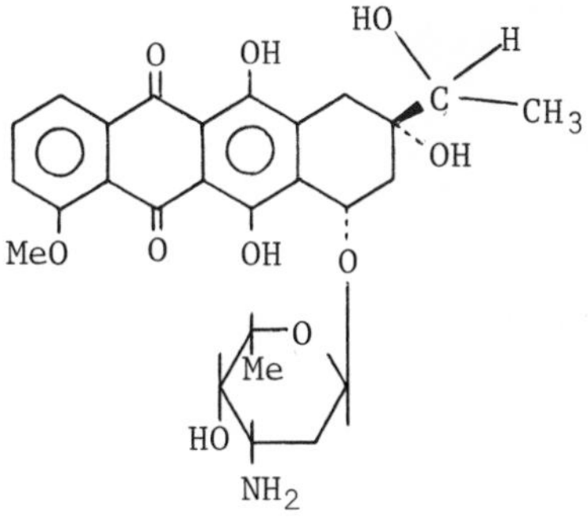

4 dihydrodaunomycin
(duborimycine)

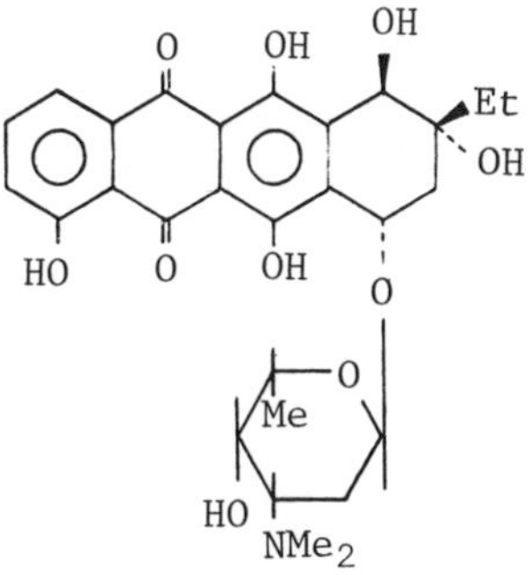

5 β-rhodomycin I
(rhodomycin B)

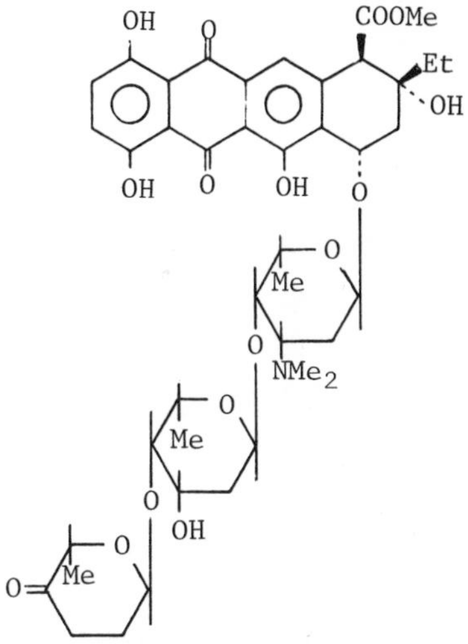

6 cinerubin A

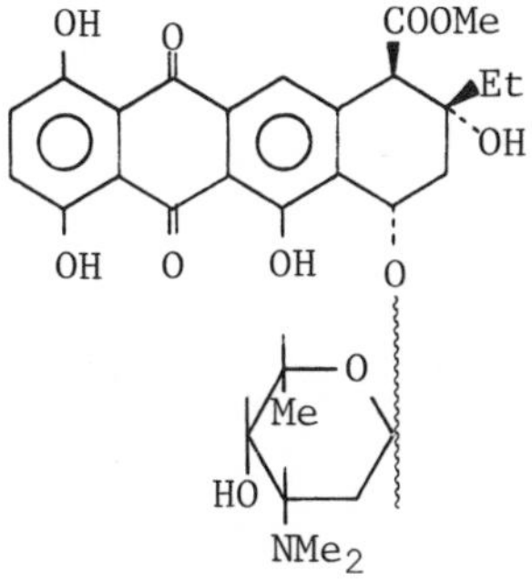

7 pyrromycin

*Figure 1. Some anthracycline antibiotics with cytotoxic activity*

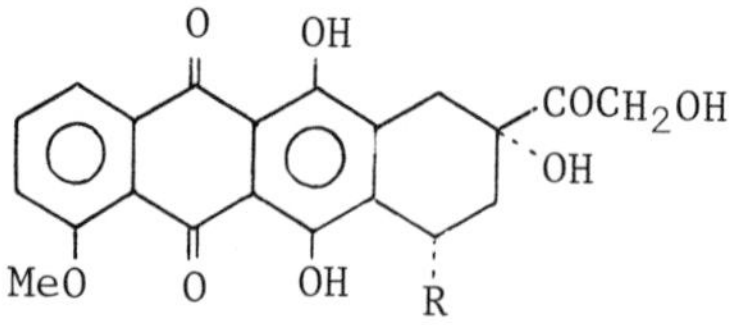

8  R = OH
9  R = H

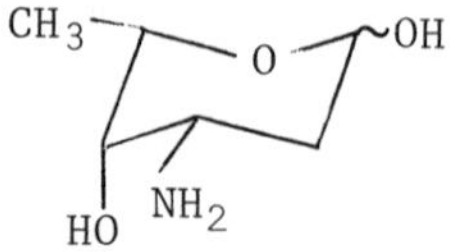

10

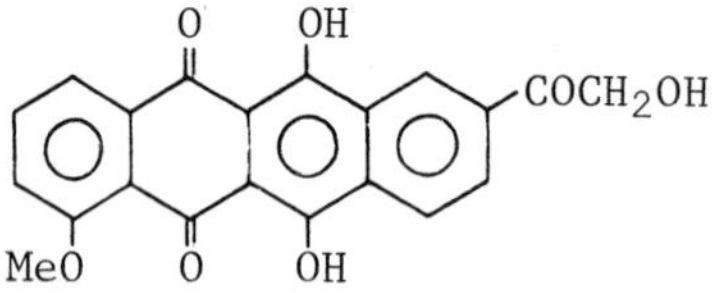

11

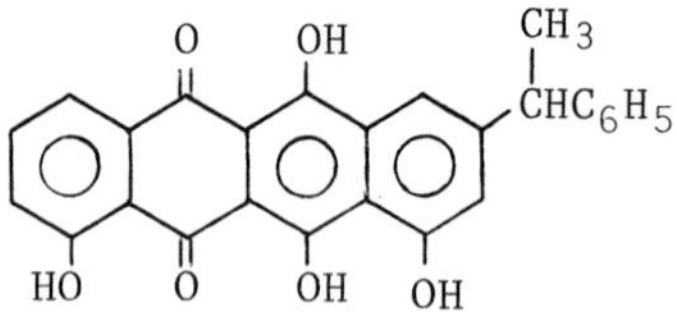

12

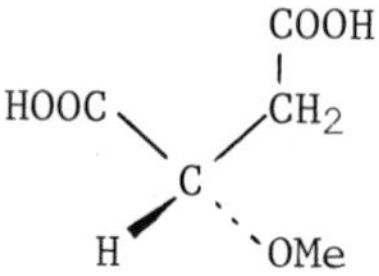

13

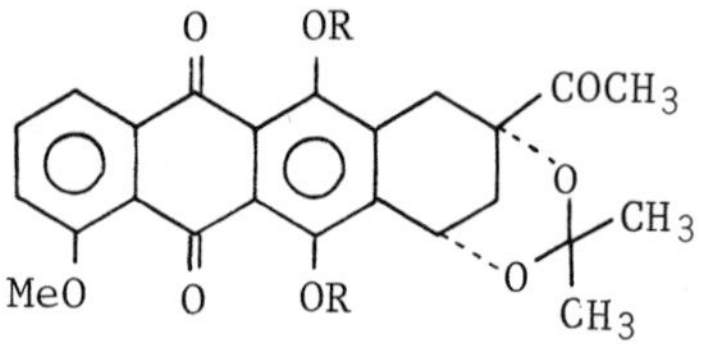

14  R = H
15  R = Me

Figure 2. Degradation products used for structure proof of adriamycin and daunomycin

The absolute stereochemistry of daunomycin followed from the isolation of carbon atoms 6a, 7, 8 and 9 as S(-)-methoxy-succinic acid (13) and the specification of a cis orientation for the 7- and 9-hydroxyls via acetonide 14. As daunosamine had been fully identified in the earlier work (24) and pmr analysis of dauno-mycin pentaacetate required the α-glycosidic configuration, these results fully characterized all chemical and steric fea-tures of the molecule. Almost simultaneously Iwamoto et al. (27) arrived at similar conclusions regarding the basic structure and relative stereochemistry of daunomycin through 220 Mc pmr spec-tral analysis of the parent antibiotic and by preparation of acetonide 15. An X-ray crystallographic analysis of N-bromo-acetyldaunomycin confirmed the assigned structure (28).

In a formal sense a total synthesis of adriamycin has been completed if the work of several groups of investigators are combined. Arcamone and his associates succeeded in converting daunomycin to adriamycin in a seven-step process in 1969 (29), thus permitting the incorporation of a daunomycin synthesis into an adriamycin synthesis. Daunosamine was first prepared from L-rhamnose in twelve steps by Marsh et al. in 1967 (30). A lengthier synthesis from glucose was reported by Yamaguchi and Kojima several years later (31). Very recently Horton and Weckerle described a high-yield process for transforming D-mannose to daunosamine (32). Daunomycinone was prepared in 1973 by Wong et al. (33). Several related studies accompanied this major accomplishment (34-37), especially noteworthy being the recent regiospecific synthesis of 9-deoxydaunomycinone by Kende et al. (38). The final segment in the total synthesis of adria-mycin was provided by Acton et al. who effected coupling of daunosamine with daunomycinone to give daunomycin (39). The syn-thesis of adriamycin provided by combining these synthetic units totals well over 40 steps; obviously there is ample opportunity for an improved route.

Clinical Results with Adriamycin. Although a full discus-sion of clinical results is beyond the scope of this paper it is appropriate to briefly note the reasons for the current intense interest in adriamycin as an antitumor drug. It is not only active against some solid tumors in man but against a wide spectrum of these tumors, many of which are poorly or non-responsive to other drugs. As a class solid tumors are most resistant to chemotherapy and past progress has been greatest in the disseminated malignancies. Table I provides selected data from a recent review by Carter and Blum on the use of adriamycin against human cancer (8). A response was defined in this study as a greater than 50% reduction in tumor mass except in the case of acute leukemia. While none of these response rates approach 100%, it is important to note that the results have been obtained in many cases from patients in which other treatments (frequently including chemotherapy) have previously failed. Regarding

Table I.    Some Human Tumors Responding
            to Adriamycin[a] .

| | | |
|---|---|---|
| Breast cancer | 36% | (44/121) |
| Sarcomas | 26% | (46/176) |
| Lung cancer | 19% | (44/229) |
| Malignant lymphomas | 41% | (61/147) |
| Acute leukemia | 24% | (47/195) |

[a]Data from ref. 8.   Numbers in parentheses
are responding patients over evaluable
patients.

adriamycin's broad spectrum of activity Carter recently reported
that adriamycin is clearly active against 9 of 19 human tumors
on which treatment statistics are satisfactory and clearly inactive in only three of them (40).   Another significant point
regarding the data in Table I is that they are based upon single-
drug treatment.   Many of the most effective chemotherapeutic
regimens for cancer are now based upon combinations of drugs,
not the use of single entities (41).   Consequently adriamycin is
currently being studied in a broad array of combination chemotherapy trials (42,43).   Among early results of these studies
Jones et al. report an 80% response rate in a group of 50 breast
cancer patients using a cyclophosphamide-adriamycin combination (44).   Gottlieb et al. have shown in a spectrum of sarcomas
that adriamycin plus 4(5)-dimethyltriazeno imidazole-5(4)-
carboxamide (DIC), with and without vincristine, provides a 50%
response rate, as opposed to a 30% response with single drugs (45).
Combined modality approaches to cancer therapy are in an early
state of development but early results here are also very promising.   Watring et al. recently reported substantial benefits by
simultaneous use of adriamycin with X-ray treatment in a small
group of patients with advanced gynecological cancers (46).
     Adriamycin is subject to the toxic side effects common to
many antitumor drugs.   Table II summarizes the incidence of the
most common toxic reactions, as reviewed by Carter and Blum (47).
Although of high frequency these effects are generally reversible
and manageable except the myocardiopathy.   This is expressed most
often as a rapidly progressing syndrome of congestive heart
failure and cardiorespiratory decompensation.   If detected early
this condition may be reversible (48) but frequently has not
responded well to treatment (49).   The cardio-toxic effects are
dose related and a cumulative dose below 500 mg/$M^2$ yields a very
low incidence of myocardiopathy (49).   In patients receiving a
greater total dose the incidence climbs rapidly and reached 30%
in one retrospective analysis (49).   Cardiotoxicity is the side
effect most limiting to the use of adriamycin at the present
time because treatment must be stopped while the tumor is still

Table II.  Incidence of Common Toxic
Effects of Adriamycin[a].

| | |
|---|---|
| Alopecia | 100% |
| Nausea/vomiting | 20-55% |
| Stomatitis | 80% |
| Leukopenia | 60-75% |
| Cardiac irregularities | |
|   EKG | 6-30% |
|   Myocardiopathy | 0.4-1.2% |

---

[a]Data from ref. 47.

responding to the drug.  The cardiotoxic character of daunomycin
is also well documented (50).

Mechanism of Action.  Di Marco and his associates have done
the majority of mechanistic studies on the anthracycline antibiotics and Arcamone and Di Marco have recently reviewed this
subject (51).  The majority of investigations in the area have
used daunomycin as the subject but many studies indicate that
adriamycin acts very similarly at the molecular level.  Both antibiotics rapidly inhibit nucleic acid synthesis in various cultured
cell lines (e.g., 52-56) and in cells of tumor bearing animals (52,57).  This phenomenon is thought to be the primary biochemical lesion caused by the drugs and to be due to selective
binding of drug to nuclear DNA.  A large body of biophysical and
biochemical data support this conclusion.  Autoradiographic
experiments clearly show, for example, that daunomycin concen-
trates in the nuclei of tumor (KB) and normal (rat liver) cells
in culture, and fluorescence quenching in drug-treated cell nuclei
also supports this contention (58).
    In vitro biophysical studies have established that daunomycin
and adriamycin form stable complexes with native DNA and that the
aglycone portion of the drugs intercalates between base pairs of
the DNA helix in the complex (51).  Characteristic alterations in
the ultraviolet and the visible spectrum of the drug (bathochromic
shift and decreased absorption) demonstrate a significant drug-DNA
association, as does a pronounced decrease of daunomycin fluorescence in the presence of DNA.  DNA alters drug chemistry as well,
inhibiting ionization of the phenolic hydroxyls at high pH and
virtually eliminating susceptibility to polarographic reduction (59,60).  Apparent binding constants for this process
($2.3-3.3 \times 10^6$ $M^{-1}$) are of the same magnitude as for the actino-
mycins, another strongly interacting group of DNA intercalating
drugs (61).  This strong binding process saturates at about one
drug molecule per five nucleotides for adriamycin and about six

nucleotides for daunomycin (60). At high drug:DNA ratios further drug binding occurs by weaker processes. Daunomycin binding to denatured DNA is reduced by a factor of 20 but the number of sites remains the same.

The properties of DNA are altered by complexation with dauno-mycin and adriamycin. As expected for intercalative binding (62, 63) the complex sediments more slowly and has a lower buoyant density than the DNA itself. The viscosity of solutions of antibiotic complexes increases with increasing drug:DNA ratios, also diagnostic for intercalative binding. In addition the drugs stabilize helical DNA to thermal denaturation, increases in melt-ing temperature ($\Delta T_m$) of 14.8° and 13.4° being observed for adria-mycin and daunomycin, respectively, in 0.01 M pH 7.0 Tris buffer at a drug:DNA ratio of 1:10 (60).

More direct evidence for the intercalative binding mechanism has also been found. Dall'acqua et al. determined by flow di-chroism experiments that the chromophores of bound daunomycin and adriamycin are perpendicular to the DNA helix axis (64). Waring demonstrated that increasing concentrations of daunomycin effect reversal of the supercoils of ØX174 closed circular DNA, a phenome-non considered highly diagnostic for intercalation (65). Pigram et al. studied fibers of DNA-daunomycin complex by X-ray diffrac-tion and concluded that the patterns obtained were consistent only with intercalative binding (66). These latter authors also pro-posed a specific molecular model for the complex in which the aglycone was largely overlapped by adjacent base pairs and the daunosamine side chain of the drug projected into the major groove of the helix with the ammonium moiety interacting ionically with a phosphate one base pair away from the intercalation site. The possibility of a hydrogen bond between the 9-hydroxy and an adja-cent phosphate was also suggested. It is of interest that dauno-mycin binds only weakly to double stranded RNA and probably by a mechanism involving only electrostatic interactions (67).

Consistent with the DNA complexing properties of these anti-biotics several investigators have reported that DNA and RNA synthesis in various isolated polymerase systems (mammalian, bacterial, viral) is inhibited by daunomycin and adriamycin and that this is due to drug-template binding rather than direct inhibition of the enzyme (56,68-72). Recent evidence suggests that adenine-thymine templates are most sensitive to transcription inhibition by daunomycin but this point is not firmly estab-lished (70).

Inhibition of viral polymerase systems, both RNA-directed (69, 72-75) and DNA-directed (76), has been investigated extensively. In one comparative study of adriamycin and daunomycin inhibition of DNA polymerases from murine sarcoma virus, rat liver and bac-teria, the viral enzyme was the most sensitive (69). The anti-biotics have been shown effective in vivo against tumors induced by murine sarcoma virus (77), Friend leukemia virus and Rous sarcoma virus (74,75).

The cell cycle phase specificities of daunomycin and adria-mycin have been investigated by several groups but general conclusions cannot yet be drawn. Tobey (78) and Kim et al. (79,80) report both antibiotics to be S-phase specific in Chinese hamster and HeLa cells, respectively. Bhuyan and Fraser concluded similarly for adriamycin in Chinese hamster fibroblasts (81). However a very detailed study by Silvestrini et al. indicated that daunomycin caused detectable inhibition of DNA and/or RNA synthesis in the $G_1$, S and $G_2$ phases of the cell cycle in rat fibroblasts (82). Mizuno et al. (71) report no phase specificity for tritiated daunomycin uptake by L-cells in contrast to the results of Silvestrini et al. (83) who found uptake maximal in the late S-phase. Mizuno et al. noted maximal cytotoxicity by daunomycin in the late S, $G_2$ and M phases but an effect was evident at all points in the cell cycle (71).

In view of the very minor structural difference between adriamycin and daunomycin, numerous investigators have sought to determine the basis for the chemotherapeutic superiority usually seen with the former (2,84). At the enzymic level Tatsumi et al. found the two drugs to be essentially equivalent as inhibitors of L1210-cell DNA polymerase (56) but Zunino and collaborators (68) found adriamycin a somewhat more potent inhibitor than daunomycin in several cell-free DNA and RNA polymerase systems. Slightly superior potency for adriamycin over daunomycin was reported earlier in viral DNA polymerase systems (69,76) but the differences are small and may vary with the template employed (74).

At the cellular level adriamycin has usually been found somewhat less potent than daunomycin when judged by criteria such as cytotoxicity, antimitotic index and inhibition of DNA synthesis, but the difference is usually quite small (54,55,79,85,86) and not always evident (57). Daunomycin is initially taken up by cells more rapidly than adriamycin however (54,56,57,87) and this absorption difference is cited by Zunino et al. (68) as the probable reason for the apparent superiority of daunomycin in L1210 cell systems. Silvestrini et al. noted that the half-life of adriamycin in Sarcoma 180 cells in mice was substantially greater than daunomycin (12 hr vs 4 hr) and that adriamycin was inhibitory to RNA synthesis in these cells at levels where daunomycin was ineffective (57). In addition these investigators found that daunomycin killed cells more quickly than adriamycin but that those cells surviving the daunomycin were capable of rapidly resuming proliferation. In contrast adriamycin had a slower cytotoxic onset but fewer cells were viable on attempted cloning after drug exposure. Razek et al. (86) also noted significant differences between the two drugs. They found AKR leukemia cells to be more sensitive to both drugs than normal hematopoietic stem cells from the mouse. However the differential toxicity between the two cell types ($TD_{50}$ normal cells/$TD_{50}$ AKR cells) for adriamycin was nearly twice as large as that for daunomycin (6.3 vs 3.6).

   One of the most significant differences between adriamycin
and daunomycin lies in the area of host immunosuppression.
Casazza et al. reported that adriamycin interfered less with the
host-mediated spontaneous regression of murine sarcoma virus
(Maloney) induced tumors than did daunomycin (88). Schwartz and
Grindey found that the substantial therapeutic advantage of adriamycin and daunomycin in treating P288 lymphocytic leukemia in mice
is lost when the host is immunosuppressed by whole-body irradiation or cyclophosphamide treatment prior to tumor implantation (87,
89). They also found that daunomycin uptake by spleen was twice
that of adriamycin whereas liver, thymus and tumor cells absorbed
the two drugs equally.
   It is clear that adriamycin and daunomycin have profound
deleterious effects on nucleic acid synthesis and this property
must be involved in their mechanism of action. However, not all
DNA-related biological effects can be directly attributed to synthesis inhibition. For example, Silvestrini et al. noted that
antimitotic effects were evident in cultured mouse cells at
daunomycin levels much too low to affect nucleic acid synthesis (82). They also demonstrated that the drug abruptly blocked
mitosis when given only a few minutes before prophase. Similarly
Schwartz recently noted that severe chromosome breakage was evident in the tumor cells of daunomycin/adriamycin treated P288-
bearing mice within 1-3 hr after treatment (90). Such breakage is
not an intrinsic property of the drug-DNA interaction however as
isolated DNA is not degraded when incubated with daunomycin (71).
   Several possible mechanisms of action for the anthracyclines
have been suggested that are apparently unrelated to DNA metabolism. Gosalvez et al. investigated the effects of adriamycin and
daunomycin on the respiration of isolated mitochondria and of
intact normal and tumor cells and found significant inhibition (91).
Similarly Folkers and co-workers determined in vitro that adriamycin, carminomycin, daunomycin and adriamycin-14-0-octanoate
inhibited succinoxidase and NADH-oxidase, respiratory chain
enzymes that require coenzyme $Q_{10}$ as cofactor (92). Comparatively
high drug levels were required to elicit these effects in both
studies. Alteration of cell surface architecture is a new effect
of adriamycin recently reported by Murphree et al. (93). Using a
new assay technique (94) they found that concanavalin A-induced
agglutination of S180 cells was enhanced severalfold following
drug exposure. As the amount of lectin bound was unchanged this
suggests that adriamycin affects the clustering of concanavalin A
binding sites.
   The possibility that adriamycin and daunomycin act by interference with microtubule function during mitosis has been raised
by the work of Dano (95,96). Induced resistance to vincristine,
vinblastine or the two anthracyclines in Ehrlich ascites tumors
was accompanied by cross-resistance to each of the others; vincristine and vinblastine are thought to act primarily on micro-
tubules.

   All of the above investigations on non-DNA-related effects
of adriamycin and daunomycin are at preliminary stages but the
possibility that these drugs act by multiple mechanisms must now
be seriously considered.

   Molecular Models.  Based upon the evidence reviewed above
(and on some data not described here) Arcamone and Di Marco (51)
concluded that DNA-adriamycin complex involves three types of
binding:  hydrophobic interaction due to the intercalated aglycone, electrostatic attraction between the protonated 3'-amino
group of the daunosamine and phosphate groups of the helix, and
hydrogen bonds of unspecified character.  The molecular model
proposed by Pigram et al. (66) for the daunomycin-DNA complex is
consistent with these conclusions.  The latter authors employed
a conformation for the daunomycin A ring similar to that found in
the crystal structure of N-bromoacetyldaunomycin (Figure 3a) (28).

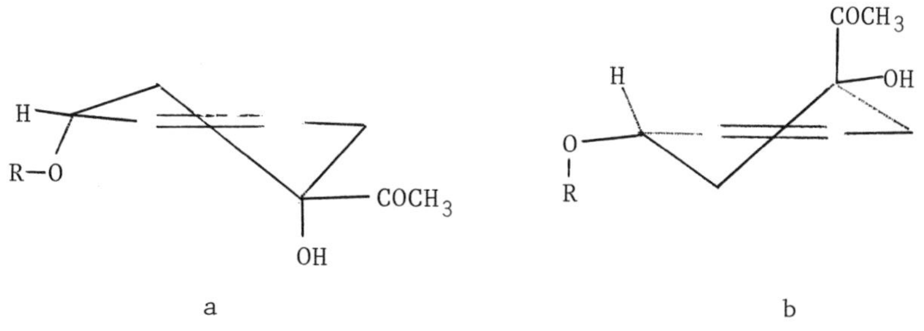

*Figure 3.   Possible conformations of ring A of daunomycin*

If another conformation of ring A is postulated (Figure 3b) a
model is possible which similarly permits the chromophore to
intercalate between base pairs and the protonated amino sugar in
the major groove to form an electrostatic bond with a DNA phosphate located one nucleotide away from the intercalation site.
However the latter conformation also clearly allows the 9-hydroxy
to hydrogen bond firmly to the phosphate adjacent to the intercalation gap and the 4'-hydroxy to probably form a hydrogen bond
to the phosphate two nucleotides away from the intercalation site.
A third hydrogen bond is possible between the 14-hydroxyl and N-7
of a purine base in the adjacent base pair.  This alternate model
complex, illustrated in Figure 4, is consistent with all of the
biophysical data and especially emphasizes the importance of the
hydrogen bonding forces that are known to contribute significantly
to the stability of the complex (97).

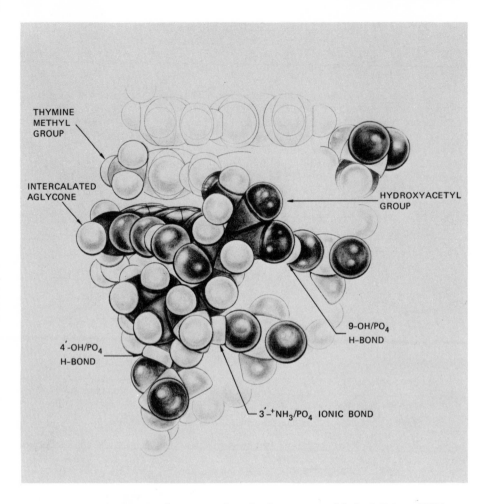

THYMINE METHYL GROUP

INTERCALATED AGLYCONE

HYDROXYACETYL GROUP

9–OH/PO$_4$ H–BOND

4′–OH/PO$_4$ H–BOND

3′–$^+$NH$_3$/PO$_4$ IONIC BOND

*Figure 4. Proposed intercalative complex of adriamycin and helical B-form DNA as viewed from the major groove. Much DNA structure has been omitted to clarify specific bonding points. Four consecutive phosphate groups from one polydeoxyribosephosphate chain are shown extending from the upper right to the lower middle positions of the drawing. The phosphate ester links in this chain are in the 3′ → 5′ direction starting from the upper right. Part of a thymine–adenine base pair is shown immediately above the aglycone. The drawing is based on a CPK molecular model.*

The drug fit in this model suggests a preference for an adenine-thymine base pair on the same side of the intercalated aglycone as the sugar residue, with the thymine located adjacent to the methoxy-bearing D-ring. However all combinations of adenine-thymine and guanine-cytosine bases around the aglycone can be accommodated except those that place the thymine toward ring A and on the same side of the molecule as the sugar residue. In these cases the thymine methyl sterically prevents formation of the ionic and hydrogen bonds associated with that region of the complex.

The alternate conformation postulated for ring A (Figure 3b) in the model of Figure 4 places the 9-acetyl group in an axial position and the 7- and 9-oxygen functions equatorial. This is contrary to the crystallographically determined conformation of N-bromoacetyldaunomycin (28) and the conformation usually found in other anthracyclinone A rings (38) (i.e., Figure 3a), thus raising the question of its probability in a DNA complex. No firm energetic justification has been made but the 3a → 3b conformational change places the large sugar moiety equatorial, possibly a not-too-unequal exchange for the axial placement of the acetyl. In addition the significant energy gain in forming the complex might be expected to more than offset any energy required to achieve the new conformation.

Overall, the proposed receptor complex pictured in Figure 4 seems satisfactory because a maximum number of drug functional groups have been used in the binding process and there are no un-filled cavities between drug and DNA or dangling parts of the drug left unused. The model offers something rare in medicinal chemistry, the opportunity to work with a reasonably possible, three-dimensional, largely chemically-defined drug-receptor structure. The concept of the specific receptor site has permeated much of drug research in recent years but full use of the idea has rarely been possible because the detailed chemical structure of the receptors are not known. Helical DNA is one of the very few bio-logical macromolecules of known importance as a drug receptor that can be described in chemical and three-dimensional terms. In the following discourse the model will be discussed in terms of its ability to rationalize test data among anthracycline derivatives and analogs.

Daunomycin and Adriamycin Derivatives. The carbonyl group at C-13 of daunomycin and adriamycin can be selectively deriva-tized by standard carbonyl reagents and, as would be expected, the amino group is also selectively attacked by acylating agents. For this reason derivatives on these functional groups received early attention in structure-activity studies (51,98). Most investigations on these classes of derivatives used daunomycin as substrate but the limited work on similar adriamycin derivatives suggests comparable effects. An important part of the data used by Arcamone and Di Marco to reach their conclusions regarding the

DNA binding mode and mechanism of action of the anthracyclines
was derived from this type of derivative (51).

In general, formation of an N-acyl derivative (amide, urea,
thiourea) of daunomycin results in a marked decrease or total
loss of in vivo antitumor activity in experimental animal screens.
Potency is always decreased markedly and usually efficacy as well.
That this is not universally so, however, is illustrated by data
on N-acetyl daunomycin (16) in Table III.  Activity against L1210
is virtually lost in this derivative but slightly superior
efficacy results in the P388 system at a higher dose.  The result
with the p-fluorophenylthiourea of adriamycin (17) in the P388
system is more typical with poorer efficacy at a high dose level
being found.  It is significant however that appreciable in vivo

Table III.  In vivo Antitumor Activity of
Adriamycin and Daunomycin Derivatives
in Three Experimental Systems[a].

| No. | Compound | % Increased survival time at optimal dose (mg/kg) | | |
|---|---|---|---|---|
| | | L1210 | P388 | B16 |
| 10 | dauno-N-COCH$_3$ | 17 (20) | 91 (12.5) 2/26C | – |
| 17 | adria-N-CSNHC$_6$H$_4$F-p | – | 50 (25) | – |
| 18 | dauno-13=NNHCOC$_6$H$_5$ | 27 (5.9) | 75 (2) | 100 (3) 1/10C[b] |
| 19 | dauno-13=NNHCOCH$_2$OH | 34 (7) | 118 (2) | 275 (6) 3/6C |
| 20 | adria-13=NNHCOC$_6$H$_5$ | – | 152 (6) 2/6C 101 (8) 1/6C | – |
| | adriamycin | 63 (1.7)[c] | 112 (1) >140 (0.5) 3/6C[b] | 94 (0.5)[b] |
| | daunomycin | 43 (1.7)[c] | 70 (0.5) 108 (0.25) | 188 (1) 4/10C[b] |

[a]Data from standard NCI mouse test systems using QD1-9 dose
schedule (99).  Fractions following entries indicate long term
survivors ("cures") over total animals in test group.  Under-
lined figures are averages of two or more values.

[b]Data from ref. 100.

[c]Data from ref. 84.

activity is retained after insertion of such a large and comparatively nonpolar group.

Carbonyl derivatization at C-13 also causes a decrease in
potency in animal tests but the effect is less than with N-
acylation and the efficacy of the derivative is occasionally
better than the parent antibiotic. Table III lists three carbonyl
derivatives. Daunomycin benzhydrazone (rubidazone, structure 18)
is equal or slightly superior to daunomycin in efficacy in the
P388 and B16 systems but 3-6 times as much drug is required for
optimum activity. In the L1210 system rubidazone appears slightly
poorer than daunomycin but it should be pointed out that both
rubidazone (and adriamycin) are schedule sensitive and the QD1-9
regimen is not optimum against L1210. With dosing every three
hours on day one after tumor implantation, for example, rubidazone
gives an increase in survival time of 61% vs 33% for daunomycin
at total doses of 32 and 4 mg/kg, respectively. On this schedule
adriamycin provides a 156% increase in survival time and two out
of eight long-term survivors at 8 mg/kg (100). Daunomycin gly-
colohydrazone (19) is clearly superior to daunomycin in the P388
and B16 systems according to the limited data available. Adriamycin benzhydrazone (20) is clearly less potent than the parent
in the one test system for which data are available but efficacy
is not seriously reduced. The data in Table III are provided to
give a general comparison of derivatives with the parent antibiotics. Detailed comparisons should be regarded with caution
because the data are not drawn from single experiments that
directly compared all compounds against each tumor.

Rubidazone (18), originally reported by Maral et al. (101),
has a greater therapeutic index than daunomycin (about two-fold)

18   rubidazone

and was evaluated against acute myeloblastic leukemia by
Jacquillat et al. (102). While a 45% complete remission rate
was achieved in this preliminary clinical study and hematological
toxicity was lessened and better controlled with rubidazone, clear
superiority over daunomycin was not established. Against solid
tumors results were less promising primarily due to unacceptable
side effects (103). Resistance to rubidazone can be induced in
the Ehrlich ascites tumor in vivo and reciprocal cross-resistance
is found with daunomycin, adriamycin, vincristine and vinblastine (104).

In vitro inhibitory effects on nucleic acid synthesis by
amino and carbonyl derivatives generally parallel their in vivo
antitumor effects, i.e., potency is almost always decreased in
comparison to the parent antibiotics. Table IV lists $ED_{50}$ values
for DNA and RNA synthesis inhibition in cultured L1210 cells for
a series of derivatives of daunomycin and adriamycin. Similar
data for several other unmodified anthracycline antibiotics are
also presented for comparison. N-Acyl derivatives usually suffer
a greater loss of potency relative to the parent than do the C-13
carbonyl derivatives. The first five compounds in Table IV were
cited in Table III for their significant in vivo antitumor activity. All of this group are inhibitory for both DNA and RNA below
10 μM but in almost every case have lost appreciable potency
relative to adriamycin and daunomycin. Derivatives 21-27 of
Table IV illustrate a different effect on DNA and RNA synthesis
that frequently results upon derivatization. The effect on DNA
synthesis is greater than it is on RNA synthesis by a factor of
three or more for each of these compounds. Daunomycin and adriamycin cause equal effects on the two types of nucleic acid under
the conditions of this assay. Since the DNA and RNA tests are
performed under identical conditions the selectivity afforded by
these compounds suggests that some aspect of their mechanism of
action has been changed by derivatization and that this effect
could be exploited to obtain drugs with favorably altered toxicity
or tumor spectrum. Three of this group of derivatives (21, 23,
25) are inactive in vivo in the L1210 or P388 systems but 22, 24,
26, and 27 retain significant activity.

It is of interest that carminomycin is the only compound encountered that showed preferential inhibition of DNA synthesis
over RNA synthesis in this system. A similar differential effect
was also noted in a bacterium (17). Rhodomycin, nogalamycin, and
the cinerubins strongly favor inhibition of RNA synthesis. The
high in vitro potency of carminomycin is reflected in its in vivo
activity. Shorin et al. (15) report somewhat superior efficacy
with carminomycin against L1210 leukemia at doses about one-
seventh those of daunomycin. These authors also report significant carminomycin activity in several other experimental tumor
systems.

An interesting class of 14-O-acyl derivatives of adriamycin
(Figure 5) was reported recently from the Farmitalia

Table IV. Inhibition of Nucleic Acid
Synthesis in Cultured L1210
Cells by Anthracycline
Antibiotics and Derivatives[a]

| No. | Compound | ED$_{50}$ ($\mu$M) DNA | RNA |
|---|---|---|---|
| 16 | dauno-N-COCH$_3$ | 7.5 | 6.8 |
| 17 | adria-N-CSNHC$_6$H$_4$F-p | 1.9 | 0.9 |
| 18 | dauno-13 = NNHCOC$_6$H$_5$ | 2.7 | 2.0 |
| 19 | dauno-13 = NNHCOCH$_2$OH | 3.5 | 2.6 |
| 20 | adria-13 = NNHCOC$_6$H$_5$ | 6.5 | 3.0 |
| 21 | dauno-N-COCH$_2$CH$_2$CH$_3$ | 66 | 21 |
| 22 | dauno-N-CSNHCH$_3$ | > 100 | 15 |
| 23 | dauno-N-CSNH(CH$_2$)$_3$CH$_3$ | 32 | 7.1 |
| 24 | dauno-N-CHO | 25 | 8.7 |
| 25 | dauno-13 = NOCH$_3$ | 2.1 | 0.7 |
| 26 | dauno-13 = NNHCO(CH$_2$)$_6$CH$_3$ | 21 | 6.5 |
| 27 | dauno-13 = NNHCOC$_6$H$_4$Et-p | 6.0 | 1.0 |
| 1 | adriamycin | 0.8 | 0.9 |
| 2 | daunomycin | 0.3 | 0.3 |
| 3 | carminomycin | 0.04 | 0.2 |
| 4 | dihydrodaunomycin | 1.2 | 2.1 |
| 5 | rhodomycin B[b] | 2.1 | 0.1 |
| – | nogalamycin[b] | 4 | 0.4 |
| 6 | cinerubin A[b] | 0.3 | 0.03 |
| – | cinerubin B[b] | 1.5 | 0.2 |

[a]Determined by drug effect on incorporation of [3]H-labeled
thymidine and uridine into DNA and RNA, respectively. ED$_{50}$
is the drug concentration effecting a 50% reduction of
labeling in isolated DNA and RNA. See ref. 105 for detailed
methodology.

[b]Antibiotics kindly provided by Dr. Martin Apple, UCSF.

Laboratories (106,107). These compounds, prepared from 14-bromo-daunomycin by displacement with carboxylate salts, frequently

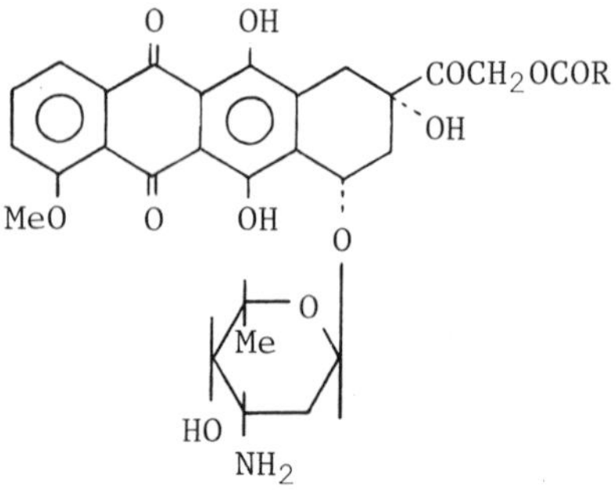

Figure 5.   Adriamycin-14-O-carboxylates prepared by Arcamone
et al. (106).  R = $CH_3$, $C_2H_5$, n-$C_7H_{15}$, $C_6H_5$, $CH_2C_6H_5$, 3-pyridyl,
$CH_2(1$-naphthyl).

displayed in vitro and in vivo cytotoxic effects comparable to adriamycin.  In some cases, notably the octanoate ester, clearly superior antitumor activity was found against Gross leukemia and transplanted mammary carcinoma in the mouse.  Pharmacokinetic studies with the octanoate demonstrate that it has altered properties relative to adriamycin; in particular the derivative accumulates in heart tissue to a smaller extent.  Preliminary data suggest that the octanoate ester is cleaved intracellularly by non-specific esterases (107).

   Another significant group of adriamycin-14-O-carboxylates was recently reported by Israel et al.  These investigators prepared a series of N-trifluoroacetylated esters (Figure 6) that showed cytotoxicity in vitro (108) and yielded one compound, N-trifluoroacetyladriamycin-14-O-valerate (code named AD32), that provided marked improvement in efficacy in their L1210 and P388 mouse leukemia systems (109).  As shown in Table V, against P388 adriamycin at 4 mg/kg gave about one-third of the survival time increase of AD32 at 40 mg/kg and no 60-day survivors.  The

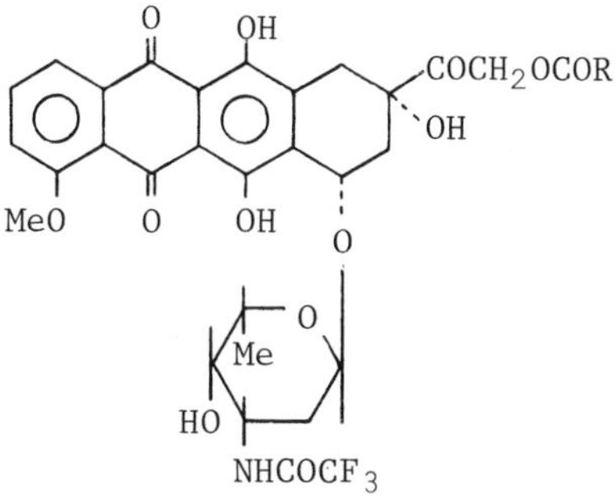

*Figure 6. N-Trifluoroacetylated adriamycin-14-O-carboxylates prepared by Israel et al. (108). R = CH₃, C₂H₅ CH(CH₃)₂, (CH₂)₃CH₃, C(CH₃)₃, (CH₂)₄CH₃, (CH₂)₆CH₃, (CH₂)₈CH₃.*

advantage of AD32 over adriamycin was even more pronounced against L1210. This tumor is intrinsically much less sensitive to anthra-cyclines and this is shown by the low survival time increase of

Table V.  Experimental Antitumor
Activity of AD32[a]

| Tumor | Drug | Optimal Dose (mg/kg) | % Increase Survival Time | 60-day Survivors |
|-------|------|----------------------|--------------------------|------------------|
| P388 | adria | 4.0 | 132 | 0/6 |
| | AD32 | 40 | 429 | 3/5 |
| L1210 | adria | 4.0 | 42 | 0/7 |
| | AD32 | 50 | > 400 | 5/7 |

[a]Schedule:  QD1-4, ip.  Data from ref. 109.

42% and lack of long-term survivors given by adriamycin.  In contrast AD32 gave five out of seven 60-day survivors, an im-pressive result as long-term survivors with any anthracycline are not common in the L1210 system.  As expected with an N-acylated derivative optimum dose levels for AD32 are at least ten-fold greater than for adriamycin.

Before leaving this group of derivatives it should be noted that their biological activities are generally in qualitative agreement with the receptor site hypothesis discussed above.

Amino, C-13 carbonyl and 14-hydroxy derivatives are all sterically acceptable according to molecular model studies. The amine
and acetyl moieties are relatively uncrowded in the complex and
can accept bulky modifications without seriously disturbing
critical binding points. The markedly decreased potencies usually
found with N-acyl derivatives are rationalized by the drug's loss
of basic character and consequent loss of the electrostatic binding component. The DNA binding constant of N-acetyldaunomycin
for example is about 200-fold less than that of daunomycin but the
number of binding sites is reduced only by one third (60).

Table VI presents two compounds that have recently emerged
from the Stanford Research Institute program (105). Periodate
treatment of adriamycin provides carboxylic acid 28 in high yield
by oxidative removal of the 14-carbon. The acid is quite poor as
a nucleic acid synthesis inhibitor in vitro but the ester (29) is

Table VI.  Biological Activity[a] of
           Periodate-modified Derivatives
           of Adriamycin

| No. | R | ED$_{50}$ (μM) | | % increase in survival time (mg/kg)[b] | ΔT$_m$ (°C)[c] |
|-----|---|------|------|-----------------------|----------|
|     |   | DNA  | RNA  |                       |          |
| 28  | OH | > 100 | 65 | 63 (25) | 2.6 |
| 29  | OCH$_3$ | 2.0 | 0.9 | 46 (50) | 12.6 |
|     | adriamycin | 0.8 | 0.9 | 112 (1) | 17.8 |

[a]See Tables III and IV for details.

[b]P388 mouse lymphocytic leukemia, QD1-9 schedule, ip tumor
  and drug.

[c]Sonicated calf thymus DNA in 0.010 M, pH 6.0 PO$_4$ buffer at a
  drug:DNA molar ratio of 1:10.

nearly as potent as adriamycin. Both compounds proved active
in vivo in the P388 system although potency and efficacy are
greatly reduced relative to adriamycin. This result is of interest none-the-less because these compounds are the first in
which the carbon skeleton of the parent has been altered with
retention of in vivo activity. There are no steric constraints
to the fit of either 28 or 29 into the proposed receptor complex
of Figure 4. However 28 is probably zwitterionic at physiological pH and the carboxylate anion would undoubtedly introduce a
strong electrostatic repulsion to the DNA phosphates and thereby
inhibit binding. This effect is reflected in the relative abilities of 28 and 29 to stabilize helical DNA. The $\Delta T_m$ of 28 is
only 2.6° vs 12.6° for ester 29 and 17.8° for adriamycin under
the standard conditions noted in Table VI.

In further new work treatment of adriamycin and daunomycin
with excess methyl iodide, followed by ion exchange, provided
quaternary ammonium chlorides (30, 31) given in Table VII (110).
DNA and RNA synthesis inhibition is greatly depressed by quaternization of both antibiotics. Reduced cell penetration because of

Table VII.  Biological Activity[a] of Quaternary
Ammonium Derivatives of Adriamycin
and Daunomycin.

| No. | R | ED$_{50}$ (μM) | | % increase in survival time (mg/kg)[b] |
|-----|---|------|------|------|
| | | DNA | RNA | |
| 30 | OH | > 100 | 83 | 90 (12.5) |
| 31 | H | > 1000 | 57 | 13 (25) |
| | adriamycin | 0.8 | 0.9 | 112 (1) |

[a] See Tables III and IV for details.

[b] P388 mouse lymphocytic leukemia, QD1-9 schedule,
ip tumor and drug.

the full and irreversible positive charge present in the drug
molecules is a probable explanation for the in vitro effect
because physical data on the daunomycin derivative indicate little
change in the binding properties with DNA.  For example, the $\Delta T_m$
for 31 is 16.3° vs 16.8° for daunomycin.  Physical data on the
adriamycin derivative are not yet available but both 30 and 31 can
be accommodated by the model receptor complex.  Surprisingly the
adriamycin quaternary retained appreciable in vivo activity while
the daunomycin derivative was inactive.  However quaternization
is clearly detrimental to in vivo activity in both cases.

Before leaving the subject of derivatives the work of Trouet
et al. on DNA complexes of daunomycin and adriamycin should be
mentioned although these materials are not derivatives in the
chemical sense used earlier in this section.  Because tumor cells
have a higher pinocytosis rate than normal cells, these investigators reasoned that complexing a drug with a macromolecular
carrier that could enter cells only by pinocytosis would result
in selective drug uptake by tumor cells.  Inside the cell subsequent lysosomal digestion of the carrier would occur and the
resulting drug release would cause cell death.  They applied this
principle, termed lysosomotropic drug action, to daunomycin and
adriamycin via the drug–DNA complexes because of the high stability of these complexes.  Although the original work (111) used
daunomycin, adriamycin–DNA complex also proved advantageous over
the free drug.  Table VIII presents comparative in vivo antitumor test data for adriamycin and its DNA complex from recent
work by Atassi and Tagnon (112).  The complex is clearly superior
to the free drug at all dose levels and induced one long-term
survivor out of ten treated animals at the highest dose.  The

Table VIII.  Activity of Adriamycin and
Adriamycin–DNA Complex Against
Leukemia L1210 in DBA/2 Mice[a]

| Dose (mg/kg)[b] | Survival time increase (%) | |
|---|---|---|
|  | Adriamycin | Adriamycin–DNA |
| 6 | 83 | 216 (1/10) |
| 5 | 141 | 216 |
| 3 | 92 | 125 |

[a]Data from ref. 112.

[b]Dose schedule QD1-5, iv.  Dose of adriamycin–DNA
complex refers to wt. of adriamycin in complex.

toxicity of the complex, based on drug content, is reduced substantially.  This type of result (113) led to successful clinical
use of daunomycin-DNA complex in the majority of patients in a
group of 25 with acute leukemias (114,115).  A favorable result
with the one patient treated with adriamycin-DNA complex was also
reported (114).  Reduced toxicity was the major advantage cited
for the complexes over the free drugs.  Additional clinical trials
with both of these promising materials are currently underway (40).
     The possibility that the role of the DNA in the adriamycin-
DNA complex is not to carry the drug into cells by endocytosis
has been raised by the work of Marks et al.  They found that DNA
injected separately before and after adriamycin, and also without
adriamycin, increased survival time in tumor bearing mice (116).

     Semisynthetic Analogs of Adriamycin and Daunomycin.  Within
the definition used in this paper two types of semisynthetic analogs are possible, those containing a natural aglycone coupled to
a daunosamine substitute and those consisting of an aglycone sur-
rogate coupled to daunosamine.  As the first examples of the
former type Penco (117) coupled daunomycinone with glucose and
glucosamine via a Koenigs-Knorr sequence to give compounds 32 and
33, respectively.  No reports on the biological properties of 32

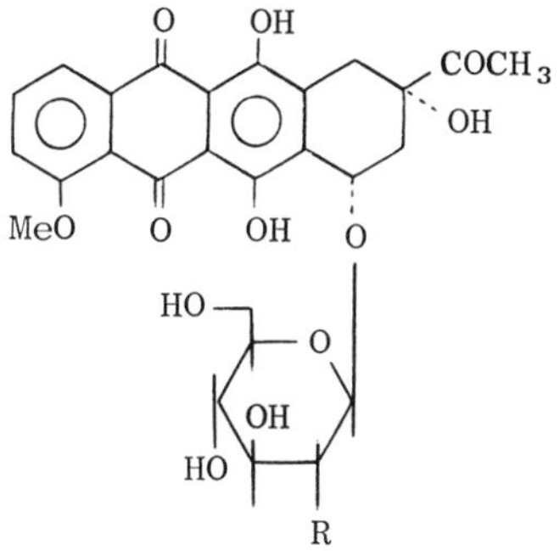

32   R = OH

33   R = NH$_2$

are known to the author but the glucosamine analog has been
studied extensively.  It binds less strongly to DNA than daunomycin (60), is less potent or inactive in a variety of in vitro
assays (77,118), and is inactive against the ascitic sarcoma 180
tumor in mice (77).  The pronounced deleterious effect of re-
placing daunosamine with glucosamine is not entirely consistent
with the molecular model of Figure 4 because an equatorial

2'-ammonium group can bond with the adjacent phosphate anion about as well as a 3'-ammonium. However, the 2'-ammonium sterically interacts with the 8-methylene of the A-ring and a conformational change in the relationship of the sugar to the A-ring could readily account for a poor fit in the hypothetical receptor complex.

Very recently the Farmitalia group (119) reported semi-synthetic analogs of daunomycin and adriamycin in which the 4'-hydroxyl is inverted with respect to the parent antibiotics (34, 35). These compounds were prepared by coupling the corresponding N,O-trifluoroacetyl-blocked chloro sugar (obtained from daunosamine) with daunomycinone and with adriamycinone, blocked at the 14-hydroxy group by a ketal. In addition to the natural α-anomers these syntheses simultaneously provided β-anomers 36 and 37 in lesser yields. The 4'-epimeric antibiotics retained roughly comparable activity to the parents as inhibitors of Murine Sarcoma

34  R = H          36  R = H
35  R = OH         37  R = OH

virus (Maloney) foci formation and mouse embryo fibroblast proliferation but appeared somewhat less potent as inhibitors of HeLa cell colony formation. In vivo 34 and 35 retained substantial activity against ascitic Sarcoma 180 and Gross leukemia in the mouse but efficacy was moderately reduced relative to the parents. 4'-Epi-adriamycin was equally efficacious but slightly less potent than adriamycin in a Sarcoma 180 solid tumor test as well. Interestingly the β-anomer of 4'-epi-daunomycin (36) retained significant activity in the various in vitro tests and against ascitic Sarcoma 180 in vivo, despite its marked configurational difference from daunomycin; potency in every test was reduced substantially in comparison with daunomycin or 34.

A very significant finding in this study was the lack of effect of 35 on the beating rate of cultured mouse embryonic heart cells at 1 μg/ml when adriamycin showed a toxic effect at 0.1 μg/ml.

This clearly demonstrates that small structural modifications can favorably affect cardiotoxic properties without destroying anti-tumor activity.

Daunomycin analogs 34 and 36 were also recently prepared at Stanford Research Institute by somewhat different methods (120, 121). Not unexpectedly we found that 4'-epi-daunomycin was essentially identical to daunomycin as an inhibitor of nucleic acid synthesis and also gave a $\Delta T_m$ value nearly as high as the parent (Table IX). The β-anomer (36) retained about one-tenth of

Table IX.  In vitro Comparison of Daunomycin
and Two Configurational Isomers.

| Compound | $ED_{50}$ (μM)[a] | | $\Delta T_m$ (°C)[b] |
|---|---|---|---|
| | DNA | RNA | |
| 34 | 0.79 | 0.24 | 15.0 |
| 36 | 6.7 | 2.9 | 5.2 |
| daunomycin | 0.80 | 0.32 | 16.8 |

[a] See Table IV for details.

[b] See Table VI for details.

of the potency of daunomycin in suppressing nucleic acid synthesis and its $\Delta T_m$ value was depressed by 11.5° below that of daunomycin. Preliminary in vivo NCI test data indicate that both 34 and 36 are active in the L1210 system.

4'-Epi-daunomycin is readily accommodated by the proposed receptor model of Figure 4 with possible loss of the 4'-hydroxyl hydrogen bond as the only change. Because of its molecular shape the β-anomer (36) cannot be fitted nearly as readily as can 34. The aglycone residue of 36 has become equatorial to the pyranose ring, rather than axial as in the α-anomers. However a reasonable conformation for 36 that permits aglycone intercalation and forma-tion of the ionic bond and the 9-hydroxy hydrogen bond can be obtained by rotation about the two carbon-oxygen bonds of the gly-cosidic link, thus qualitatively rationalizing the decreased potency and $\Delta T_m$.

Structure 38 is another semisynthetic analog derived from daunomycinone (122). In this compound the daunosamine moiety is replaced by the basic but much simpler β-alanine ester function. Because of the flexibility of the acyclic β-alanine side chain this compound can readily be accommodated by the receptor model. Compared to daunomycin 38 inhibits DNA and RNA synthesis in cultured L1210 cells at about ten-fold higher levels ($ED_{50}$ = 8.2 and 5.7 μM, respectively). In vivo antitumor activity was also

38

found with this compound, giving increases in survival time in two
tests of 60 and 26% at 12.5 mg/kg and 69 and 26% at 6.25 mg/kg
(P388, QD1-9 ip regimen). The $\Delta T_m$ value for 38 under our standard conditions (Table VI) was reduced but significant at 6.3°.
Although the in vivo activity of 38 is unremarkable compared to
adriamycin and daunomycin it reinforces the conclusion suggested
previously by the properties of 34-36 that daunosamine provides
nothing irreplaceable in the anthracycline antibiotics and may
simply be a carrier for a potency-enhancing ammonium moiety. This
point will be considered further in following discussions.

Several esters of daunomycinone analogous to 38 but derived
from amine-bearing cyclohexane carboxylic acids have been patented
and claimed as effective against L1210 lymphocytic leukemia in the
mouse (123).

Moving to the second type of semisynthetic analog, Table X
presents a series of glycosides of daunosamine with a variety of
synthetic aglycones (124). These compounds are part of a series
designed to determine what features of the natural aglycones are
essential for biological activity. Deleting all aromatic character and retaining only ring A of daunomycinone provided 39. Virtually all activity as an inhibitor of DNA and RNA synthesis in
cell culture is lost by this simplification. The $\Delta T_m$ value for
39 has not been determined but a low value would be expected
because intercalation is impossible with no aromatic group.
Coupling of daunosamine to α-tetralol, thus reinstating a little
aromatic character in the aglycone, yielded the diastereomeric
pair, 40 and 41. Neither compound displayed significant DNA/RNA
synthesis inhibition nor provided $\Delta T_m$ values appreciably above
baseline (i.e., no better than daunosamine). Extension of the
aromatic area of the series by use of biphenyl-4-carbinol as
aglycone provided compound 42. A nearly ten-fold enhancement of
nucleic acid synthesis inhibition results from this change but the
ability of the compound to thermally stabilize DNA remains insignificant. Moving to anthraquinone-2-carbinol as aglycone, thus
adding a third aromatic ring and quinonoid character to the system,
provided analog 43. All activity parameters improved; DNA and RNA
synthesis inhibition values fell below 10 μM and the $\Delta T_m$ rose to
the low but significant value of 2.2°. Coupling daunosamine to a
simplified tetrahydronaphthacene quinone analog of daunomycinone
that was prepared previously in our laboratories (37,125) yielded

the diasteriomeric pair of analogs 44 and 45.  Compound 44 now
resembles the parent antibiotics quite closely, possessing a
chromophore with very similar electronic character, correct
stereochemistry at the 7-position and only lacking the 9-position
substituents and the 4-methoxy group.  These seeming advances
toward the parent antibiotics improved the DNA/RNA inhibitory
character of the drug somewhat but by a factor of less than two
over anthraquinone 43.  On the other hand the $\Delta T_m$ value for 44
rose quite significantly to 12.6°.  Perhaps most importantly,
however, the diastereomer of unnatural R configuration at the 7-
position (45) was as good an inhibitor of nucleic acid synthesis
as was 44 despite their marked stereochemical difference.  The
$\Delta T_m$ of 45 also improved over the simpler analogs but much less so
than that of 44.

The $\Delta T_m$ data are consistent with the receptor site model
given in Figure 4.  For maximum stability of the complex the drug
should possess an aromatic component that permits maximum overlap
with the surrounding base pairs.  This condition is met with the
analogs showing significant $\Delta T_m$ values.  In addition, the correct
configuration at the 7-position combined with the largest aromatic moiety (compound 44) yielded the highest DNA stabilization
seen in the series.  The nucleic acid synthesis inhibition values
also correlate generally with what the model would predict:
structural features expected to give a more stable complex are
associated with greater inhibitory effects.  However compound 45
is an important exception to this generalization.  The inversion
of the benzylic carbon (equivalent to C-7 of adriamycin) yields a
molecule that essentially cannot participate in the hypothetical
receptor site.  The molecular shape of 45 differs sharply from
that of 44; the latter fits into the site as easily as adriamycin
(less the 9- and 14-hydroxy hydrogen bonds) while 45 can be made
to fit only poorly by assuming improbable conformations.  Although
it is possible according to model studies for analog 45 to form
ionically bound intercalative complexes with DNA that differ substantially from that of Figure 4, adriamycin and daunomycin cannot
be accommodated.  Thus the similar $ED_{50}$ values for 44 and 45
could be caused fortuitously by a unique DNA complex assumed by
45, but not by the antibiotics.  However the data seem better
rationalized by the proposition that adriamycin, daunomycin, 45
and all of the in vitro-active analogs can affect nucleic acid
synthesis by an alternate and comparatively nonstereospecific
mechanism in addition to the single specific mechanism implied by
the molecular complex pictured in Figure 4.

All analogs in Table X except 39 have been evaluated in vivo
by NCI in the P388 system.  All were found inactive at non-toxic
doses.  The lack of in vivo activity from any of the analogs,
especially 44, implies that one or more of the 4- and 9-position
substituents of adriamycin and daunomycin are necessary for a
useful drug.  The DNA/RNA synthesis inhibition shown by 44, while
not as potent as that of the parents, is well within the range

Table X. Glycosides of Daunosamine. Inhibition of Nucleic Acid Synthesis in Cultured L1210 Cells and Effect on Thermal Denaturation of Calf Thymus DNA.

| No. | R | ED$_{50}$ ($\mu$M)[a] | | $\Delta T_m$ (°C)[b] |
|-----|---|------|------|------|
| | | DNA | RNA | |
| 39 | (diastereomeric mixture) | 210 | 210 | – |
| 40 | | 220 | 210 | 0.5 |
| 41 | | 280 | 210 | 0.9 |
| 42 | | 28 | 28 | 1.1 |

Table X (Concluded)

| No. | R | ED$_{50}$ ($\mu$M)[a] | | $\Delta T_m$ (°C)[b] |
|---|---|---|---|---|
| | | DNA | RNA | |
| 43 | | 9.0 | 7.4 | 2.2 |
| 44 | | 5.6 | 4.7 | 12.6 |
| 45 | | 5.4 | 4.5 | 6.8 |
| | adriamycin | 0.8 | 0.9 | 17.8 |
| | daunomycin | 0.3 | 0.3 | 16.8 |
| | daunosamine | > 100 | > 100 | 1.0 |

[a] See Table IV for details.

[b] See Table VI for specific conditions.

where useful in vivo-active derivatives appear (see Tables III
and IV). This suggests that the need for these additional substituents may lie in the realm of host effects rather than in
their importance for increasing intrinsic tumor-cell killing
character.

    Totally Synthetic Analogs of Adriamycin.  Analogs of this
group are associated with the anthracycline natural products
primarily by possessing two structural features in common,
a quininoid aromatic unit and a basic side chain.  Analogs of
this type were first described by Muller et al. (126) who prepared
racemic 46 and several other related compounds as analogs of
rhodomycin B and daunomycin.  No data on the biological or biophysical properties of these compounds have yet been published
however.
    Very recently Double and Brown (127) prepared a series of
five anthraquinones bearing one or two aminoalkylamino side chains
(e.g., 47-49) as models of several intercalating drugs including

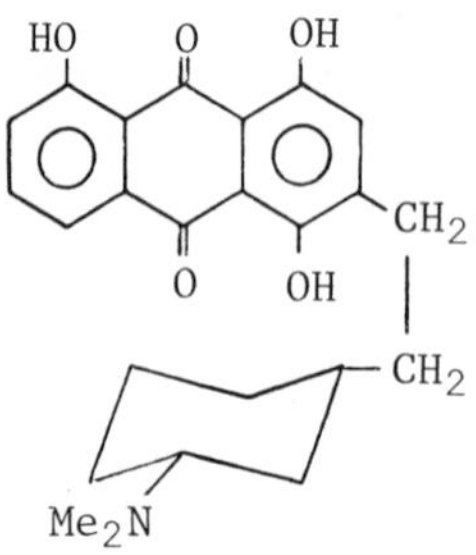

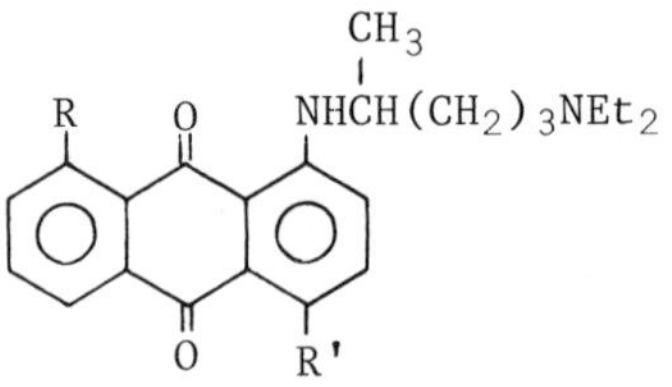

47   R = H,  R' = OH

48   R = H,  R' = NHCH(CH$_2$)$_3$NEt$_2$
              CH$_3$

49   R = NHCH(CH$_2$)$_3$NEt$_2$,  R' = H
          CH$_3$

46

adriamycin.  Spectrophotometric DNA-binding studies determined
that compounds 47 and 48 had binding constants slightly greater
than adriamycin but that the number of receptor sites on the DNA
was reduced by 25-50%.  Compound 49 possessed a binding constant
about one-half that of adriamycin but the apparent number of
receptor sites was equivalent to the antibiotic.  No biological
data on these compounds have been published but it is significant
that such relatively accessible and simple analogs exhibit DNA
binding characteristics very similar to those of the much more
complex parent antibiotics.

Racemic β-alanine ester 50 was prepared by Yamamoto et al. (128) and is a close relative of corresponding daunomycinone ester 38. This compound inhibits DNA and RNA synthesis in cultured L1210 cells with $ED_{50}$ values of 2.6 and 2.8 μM, respectively. These values are only three-fold higher than adriamycin in

50

the same test and severalfold less than those of 38. The $\Delta T_m$ value for 50 is 5.2° compared to 17.8° for adriamycin and 6.3° for 38 under similar conditions (see Table VI). Analog 50 was inactive in vivo in the standard L1210, P388 and B16 tests. The high in vitro potency of 50, despite its considerable structural deviation from adriamycin and daunomycin, provides additional encouragement that simplified analogs can possess the necessary cytotoxicity. The lack of in vivo activity of 50 when compared to 38 emphasizes again the apparent importance of one or more of the 4- and 9-substituents in attempting to reproduce the therapeutic characteristics of the natural products in less complex molecules.

Table XI presents three fully aromatic dihydroxynaphthacenequinones bearing basic substituents that may be regarded as analogs of adriamycin. Compound 51 was reported by Finkelstein and Romano (129) to have in vivo activity against Sarcoma 180 and solid Ehrlich carcinoma tumors but no activity was seen in the L1210 and P388 systems of the NCI. Believing that a longer, more basic side chain would confer greater similarity to daunomycin, basic amides 52 and 53 were prepared from 51 (130). The N,N-diethylglycyl side chain of 52 provided no improvement over 51 as an inhibitor of nucleic acid synthesis or in vivo. The longer, N,N-diethyl-β-alanyl, homolog (53) was detectably active in the in vitro test but significant activity against L1210 and P388 in vivo was not seen. DNA melting temperature measurements on 51-53 were not possible because of water insolubility.

Table XI.   5,12-Dihydroxynaphthacene-6,11-diones
as Inhibitors of Nucleic Acid Synthesis.[a]

| No. | Structure | ED$_{50}$ (µM) DNA | RNA |
|-----|-----------|-----|-----|
| 51 | O OH / O OH NH$_2$ | > 100 | > 100 |
| 52 | O OH / O OH NHCOCH$_2$NEt$_2$ | > 100 | > 100 |
| 53 | O OH / O OH NHCOCH$_2$CH$_2$NEt$_2$ | 49 | 39 |
| | adriamycin | 0.8 | 0.9 |

[a] See Table IV for details.

In Table XII are presented two N-substituted-1-amino-4-hydroxyanthraquinone that may be regarded as tricyclic analogs of adriamycin (131). Both display moderate levels of nucleic acid synthesis inhibition and substantial thermal stabilization of DNA. Compound 54 is essentially a lower homolog of 47, one of the compounds described by Double and Brown (127) as binding to DNA with a constant equal to adriamycin. Compound 54 has shown marginal but confirmed activity against P388 lymphocytic leukemia in the mouse in the QD1-9 schedule (ca 25% increase in survival time at

Table XII. 1-Amino-4-hydroxyanthraquinones.
Inhibition of Nucleic Acid Synthesis
in Cultured L1210 Cells and Effect on
Thermal Denaturation of Calf Thymus DNA.

| No. | Structure | $ED_{50}$ ($\mu$M)[a] | | $\Delta T_m$ (°C)[b] |
|-----|-----------|------|------|------|
| | | DNA | RNA | |
| 54 | | 8.2 | 6.7 | 12.4 |
| 55 | | 19 | 15 | 10.6 |
| | adriamycin | 0.8 | 0.9 | 17.8 |

---

[a] See Table IV for details.

[b] See Table VI for specific conditions.

50–100 mg/kg) but was inactive against L1210. In vivo assays on 55 have not been obtained.

The last group (132) of totally synthetic analogs, listed in Table XIII, is characterized by a variety of basic side chains in the 2-position of the aromatic nucleus. The compounds with 1,4-dihydroxyanthraquinone nuclei and aliphatic side chains (56, 57) were significantly inhibitory in the in vitro test but the presence of a phenyl ring in the side chain destroyed all activity (58, 59). The presence of a phenyl in a basic side chain on the 1-position (55, Table XII) was much less detrimental to in vitro activity.

The last three compounds of Table XIII, all incorporating naphthoquinone rings, are the most remote from the anthracycline antibiotics of all analogs prepared. Appreciable DNA/RNA synthesis inhibition was nevertheless encountered, especially with 62. The possibility must be considered that these highly

Table XIII.  2-Substituted Anthraquinones and
Naphthoquinones as Inhibitors of
Nucleic Acid Synthesis in Cultured
L1210 Cells.[a]

| No. | Structure | $ED_{50}$ ($\mu$M) | |
| --- | --- | --- | --- |
| | | DNA | RNA |
| 56 | | 19 | 8 |
| 57 | | 18 | 14 |
| 58 | | > 100 | > 100 |
| 59 | | > 100 | > 100 |
| 60 | | 20 | 23 |
| 61 | | 39 | 35 |
| 62 | | 6.1 | 6.5 |
| | adriamycin | 0.8 | 0.9 |

[a] See Table IV for details.

simplified compounds are acting through a totally different
mechanism since the intercalating potential of the naphthalene
ring is decreased because of its smaller size. $\Delta T_m$ data are not
available on all compounds but 60 and 61 provided values of only
1.5° under our standard conditions.

All analogs in Table XIII were inactive at non-toxic doses
in the P388 and L1210 systems. Naphthoquinone 62 was notable for
its high toxicity, causing a high proportion of early deaths among
treated mice at doses above 1.5 mg/kg on the QD1-9 schedule.

All analogs in Tables XI-XIII are structurally capable of
intercalating into DNA with the basic side chains forming ionic
bonds with adjacent phosphates. However the lack of side chain
and aglycone optical asymmetry and the conformational flexibility
of the side chains make it difficult to draw useful conclusions
relative to the proposed adriamycin-DNA receptor complex discussed
earlier. These molecules can participate in a spectrum of possible binding modes according to molecular model studies and no
obvious advantage can be assigned to any one of them.

It is significant that DNA binding parameters comparable to
those of adriamycin and daunomycin are found with these much-
simplified analogs and that substantial DNA and RNA synthesis
inhibitory character frequently parallels this behaviour. While
data are inadequate to firmly associate their mechanism of action
with that of adriamycin, their comparatively ready synthetic
accessibility coupled with their frequently interesting effects
on nucleic acid synthesis make them a class of compounds with good
prospects for yielding a useful antitumor drug. The in vivo
activity found for 54 further supports this suggestion.

Conclusions. The most obvious conclusion to be drawn from
the foregoing discussion is that it is difficult to improve on
Nature. In only a few instances have structural manipulations
with adriamycin or daunomycin provided superior efficacy, and in
no case has superior potency resulted. Yet, improved properties
appear to have occasionally resulted from structures such as
rubidazone (18), AD32 (Figure 6), 4'-epi-adriamycin (35), and
the antibiotic-DNA complexes (Table VIII). Further research at
the preclinical and clinical level will be necessary to fully
reveal the value of these materials for human therapy.

To date in vivo antitumor activity has been associated almost
exclusively with derivatives and analogs that have carbon skeletons identical to those of adriamycin and daunomycin. The most
efficacious modifications have been obtained by derivatization of
the parent antibiotics (e.g., Table III) or by a small stereochemical change as in the 4'-epimeric antibiotics (34 and 35).
The work with the daunosamine glycosides (Table X) and the β-
alanyl esters (38 and 50) suggest that optimum in vivo activity
is related to the presence of one or more of the 4- and 9-
substituents. Yet appreciable, if not remarkable, in vivo
activity has been displayed by compounds with skeletons deviating

significantly from those of the parents (28, 29, 38), thus
providing encouragement that there is no absolute requirement
for the native skeleton and other skeletal variants could offer
better antitumor properties and decreased toxicity.  The number
of possible structural parameters of adriamycin potentially subject to investigation is very large and only a few have been
approached, due primarily to the difficult chemistry of the
anthracyclines.  This situation will, unquestionably, change in
the future because of the accelerating therapeutic interest in
adriamycin.

The breadth of structural types showing significant inhibitory effects on nucleic acid synthesis in cell culture is much
greater than that showing in vivo antitumor action.  While it is
well known that in vitro systems characteristically provide positive results more frequently than whole-animal tests, the structural spectrum yielding  $ED_{50}$  values below 10 μM is nevertheless
very broad.  Whether the most structurally remote compounds
(e.g., 62) are truly related to adriamycin, or serendipitously
act by different mechanisms, the potential for developing in vivo
antitumor activity from them seems high because they are readily
approached synthetically and structural parameters can be easily
altered.

Perhaps the most valuable result from the derivative and
analog work reviewed here will be separation of antitumor activity from cardiotoxicity.  Until recently very little was known
about the relation of chemical structure to cardiotoxicity (133,
134) because no animal models for this syndrome were available.
Several test systems have been reported recently (135-138) and
cardiotoxicity evaluations may be expected to become an essential
part of analog evaluation.  The favorably altered effects of 4'-
epi-adriamycin (35) when compared to adriamycin was previously
noted (119).

The DNA binding site hypothesis cited throughout the discussion has been a fascinating tool for the study of adriamycin
analogs.  It has provided a conceptual base on which to evaluate
the effects of structural changes on biophysical and biological
properties of drug candidates but has not yet provided any unique
insights that have led to design of improved drugs.  The latter
point is not too surprising in view of our incomplete knowledge
on the state of DNA in the nucleus of living cells; many factors
in addition to receptor fit must govern the effect of a drug on
the complexities of DNA function.  On the other hand, the physical data that were obtained by Di Marco and colleagues (51) on
the binding of daunomycin derivatives and analogs to isolated
DNA, as well as our $\Delta T_m$ measurements, are consistent with the
model.  Structural changes that delete or decrease the various
binding forces maintaining the complex result in destabilization.
The divergence of the biological properties of analogs such as 45
from their DNA binding properties can thus be interpreted as evidence that the mechanism of action of the anthracycline

Antibiotics does not involve a single stereospecific receptor. Future structure-activity work will undoubtedly shed more light on this point.

Some of the concepts described in this paper were briefly discussed in an earlier symposium report (139).

Acknowledgment. The author gratefully acknowledges the work of Dorris Taylor and Brenda Williamson who ably performed the nucleic acid synthesis inhibition assays and DNA binding studies. Thanks are due also to Dr. Harry B. Wood, Jr. of the Division of Cancer Treatment, NCI, for suggestions and helpful discussions. Supported by Contract No. 1-CM-33742 from the Division of Cancer Treatment, NCI, NIH, USPHS.

## Literature Cited

1. Arcamone, F., Cassinelli, G., Fantini, G., Grein, A., Orezzi, P., Pol, C., and Spalla, C.  Biotechnology and Bioengineering (1969), 11, 1101.
2. Di Marco, A., Gaetani, M., and Scarpinato, B.  Cancer Chemo. Rpts. (1969), 53, 33.
3. Cassinelli, G., Orezzi, P., and Gior, P.  Microbiol. (1963), 11, 167.
4. Dubost, M., Ganter, P., Maral, R., Ninet, L., Pinnert, S., Preud'homme, J., and Werner, S. H.  C. R. Acad. Sci. (Paris) (1963), 257, 1813.
5. Brachnikova, M. G., Kostantinova, N. V., Pomaskova, P. A., and Zacharov, B. M.  Antibiotiki (1966), 11, 763.
6. Daunomycin, Chemotherapy Fact Sheet.  Published by Program Analysis Branch, National Cancer Institute, Bethesda, Md. 20014, March 1970.
7. "Recent Results in Cancer Research. Rubidomycin," Bernard, J., Paul, R., Boiron, M., Jacquillat, Cl., and Maral, R., eds., Springer-Verlag, New York, 1969.
8. Blum, R. H. and Carter, S. K.  Ann. Internal Med. (1974), 80, 249.
9. Skovsgaard, F. and Nissen, N. I.  Danish Med. Bull. (1975), 22, 62.
10. Bonadonna, G., Beretta, G., Tancini, G., De Palo, G. M., Gasparini, M., and Doci, R.  Tumori (1974), 60, 373.
11. Brockmann, H.  Prog. Chem. Org. Nat. Prods. (1963), 21, 121.
12. Thomson, R. H.  "Naturally Occurring Quinones," 2nd ed., pp 536-575, Academic Press, London, 1971.
13. Gauze, G. F., Sveshnekova, M. A., Ukholina, R. S., Gavenlina, G. V., Filicheva, V. A., and Gladkikh, E. G.  Antibiotiki (1973), 18, 675.
14. Brazhnikova, M. G., Zbarsky, V. B., Kudinova, M. K., Murav'eva, L. I., Ponomarenko, V. I., and Potapova, N. P.  Antibiotiki (1973), 18, 678.

15. Shorin, V. A., Bazhanov, V. S., Averbuch, L. A., Lepeshkiner, G. N., and Girinshtein, A. M.  Antibiotiki (1973), 18, 681.
16. Brazhnikova, M. G., Zbarsky, V. B., Potapova, N. P., Sheinker, Yu. N., Vlasova, T. F., and Rozynov, B. V. Antibiotiki (1973), 18, 1059.
17. Dudnik, Yu. V., Ostanina, L. N., Kozmyan, L. I., and Gauze, G. G.  Antibiotiki (1974), 19, 514.
18. Vertogradova, T. P., Gol'dberg, L. E., Filippos'yants, S. T., Belova, I. P., Stepanova, E. S., and Shepelevtseva, N. G. Antibiotiki (1974), 19, 50.
19. Gol'dberg, L. E., Filippos'yants, S. T., Kunrat, I. A., Stepanova, E. S., and Shepelevtseva, N. G.  Antibiotiki (1974), 19, 57.
20. Brazhnikova, M. G., Zbarsky, V. B., Ponomarenko, V. I., and Potapova, N. P.  J. Antibiotics (1974), 27, 254.
21. Gause, Georgij F., Brazhnikova, Maria G., and Shorin, Vitalif A.  Cancer Chemo. Rpts., Part 1 (1974), 58, 255.
22. Arcamone, F., Franceschi, G., Penco, S., and Selva, A. Tetrahedron Letters (1969), 1007.
23. Arcamone, F., Franceschi, G., Orezzi, P., Cassinelli, G., Barbieri, W., and Mondelli, R.  J. Am. Chem. Soc. (1964), 86, 5334.
24. Arcamone, F., Cassinelli, G., Orezzi, P., Franceschi, G., and Mondelli, R.  J. Am. Chem. Soc. (1964), 86, 5335.
25. Arcamone, F., Franceschi, G., Orezzi, P., Penco, S., and Mondelli, R.  Tetrahedron Letters (1968), 3349.
26. Arcamone, F., Cassinelli, G., Franceschi, G., Orezzi, P., and Mondelli, R.  Tetrahedron Letters, (1968), 3353.
27. Iwamoto, R. H., Lim, P., and Bhacca, N. S.  Tetrahedron Letters (1968), 3891.
28. Angiuli, R., Foresti, E., Riva di Sanseverino, L., Isaacs, N. W., Kennard, O., Motherwell, W.D.S., Wampler, D. L., and Arcamone, F.  Nature New Biology (1971), 234, 78.
29. Arcamone, F., Barbieri, W., Franceschi, G., and Penco, S. Chim. Ind. (Milan) (1969), 51, 834.
30. Marsh, J. P., Mosher, C. W., Acton, E. M., and Goodman, L. Chem. Comm. (1967), 973.
31. Yamaguchi, T. and Kojima, M.  Abstr. Symp. on the Chemistry of Natural Products, Tokyo, 1973, p 205.
32. Horton, Derek and Weckerle, Wolfgang.  Abstr. 170th Nat. Meeting Am. Chem. Soc., Chicago, Ill, August 25-29, 1975. Abstr. CARB 4.
33. Wong, C. M., Schwenk, R. Popien, D., and Ho, T.-L.  Can. J. Chem. (1973), 51, 466.
34. Wong, C. M., Popien, D., Schwenk, R., and Te Raa, J.  Can. J. Chem. (1971), 49, 2712.
35. Horii, Z., Ozaki, Y., Yamamura, S., Hanaoka, M., and Momose, T.  Chem. Pharm. Bull. (1971), 19, 2200.
36. Horii, Z., Ozaki, Y., Yamamura, S., Nishikado, T., Hanaoka, M., and Momose, T.  Chem. Pharm. Bull. (1974), 22, 93.

37. Marsh, J. P., Iwamoto, R. H., and Goodman, L. Chem. Comm. (1968), 589.
38. Kende, A. S., Belletiere, J., Bentley, T. J., Hume, E., and Airey, J. J. Am. Chem. Soc. (1975), 97, 4425.
39. Acton, E. M., Fujiwara, A. N., and Henry, D. W. J. Med. Chem. (1974), 17, 659.
40. Carter, S. K. "Adriamycin - Thoughts for the Future." Presentation at the Fifth New Drug Seminar, DCT, NCI, Dec. 16-17, 1974, Wash., D.C.
41. De Vita, V. T., Young, R. C., and Canellos, G. P. Cancer (1975), 35, 1.
42. Carter, S. K. and Blum, R. H., 1974 Report of the Division of Cancer Treatment, NCI, NIH, DHEW, Vol. 2, Sept. 1974, pp 7.170-7.186.
43. Bonadonna, Gianni et al. Tumori (1974), 60, 393.
44. Jones, S. E., Durie, B.G.M., and Salmon, S. E. Cancer (1975), 36, 90.
45. Gottlieb, J. A., Baker, L. H., O'Bryan, R. M., Luce, J. K., Sinkovics, J. G., and Quagliana, J. M. Biochem. Pharmacol. Suppl. No. 2, (1974), 183-192.
46. Watring, W. G. et al. Gynecol. Oncol. (1974), 2, 518.
47. Carter, S. K. and Blum, R. H. Ca (1974), 24, 322.
48. Gilladoga, A. C., Tan, C., Wollner, N., Murphy, M., and Sternberg, S. Proc. Am. Assoc. Can. Res. (1973), 14, 95.
49. Lefrak, E. A., Pitha, J., Rosenheim, S., and Gottlieb, J. Cancer (1973), 32, 302.
50. Buja, L. M., Ferrans, V. J., Mayer, R. J., Roberts, W. C., and Henderson, E. S. Cancer (1973), 32, 771 and references cited therein.
51. Di Marco, A. and Arcamone, F. Arzneimittel Forsch. (1975), 25, 368.
52. Theologides, A., Yarbro, J. W., and Kennedy, B. J. Cancer (1968), 21, 16.
53. Rusconi, A. and Di Marco, A. Cancer Res. (1969), 29, 1507.
54. Meriwether, W. D. and Bachur, N. R. Cancer Res. (1972), 32, 1137.
55. Dano, K., Frederiksen, S., and Hellung-Larsen, P. Cancer Res. (1972), 32, 1307.
56. Tatsumi, K., Nakamura, T., and Wakisaka, G. Gann (1974), 65, 237.
57. Silvestrini, R., Lenaz, L., Di Fronzo, G., and Sanfilippo, O. Cancer Res. (1973), 33, 2954.
58. "Rubidomycin," Bernard, J., Paul, R., Boiron, M., Jacquillat, Cl., and Maral, R., eds., pp 46-47, Springer-Verlag, New York, 1969.
59. Calendi, E., Di Marco, A., Reggiani, M., Scarpinato, B., and Valentini, L. Biochim. Biophys. Acta (1965), 103, 25.
60. Zunino, F., Gambetta, R., Di Marco, A., and Zaccara, A. Biochim. Biophys. Acta (1972), 277, 489.

61. Muller, W. and Crothers, D. M.   J. Mol. Biol. (1968), 35, 251.
62. Lerman, L. S.   J. Mol. Biol. (1961), 3, 18.
63. Lerman, L. S.   J. Cell and Compar. Physiol. (1964), 64, Supp. 1, 1.
64. Dall'acqua, F., Terbojevich, M., Marciani, S., Vedaldi, D., and Rodighiero, G.   Il Farmaco, Ed. Sci. (1974), 29, 682.
65. Waring, Michael.   J. Mol. Biol. (1970), 54, 247.
66. Pigram, W. J., Fuller, W., and Hamilton, L. D.   Nature New Biol. (1972), 235, 17.
67. Doskocil, J. and Fric, I.   FEBS Lett. (1973), 37, 55.
68. Zunino, F., Gambetta, R., and Di Marco, A.   Biochem. Pharma- col. (1975), 24, 309.
69. Zunino, F., Gambetta, R., Di Marco, A., Zaccara, A., and Luoni, G.   Cancer Res. (1975), 35, 754.
70. Zunino, F., Di Marco, A., Zaccara, A., and Luoni, G.   Chem.-Biol. Interactions (1974), 9, 25 and references cited therein.
71. Mizuno, N. S., Zakis, B., and Decker, R. W.   Cancer Res. (1975), 35, 1542.
72. Ward, D. C., Reich, E., and Goldberg, I. H.   Science (1965), 149, 1259.
73. Apple, M. A. and Haskell, C. M.   Physiol. Chem. & Phys. (1971), 3, 307.
74. Chandra, P., Zunino, F., Gotz, A., Gericke, D., Thorbeck, R., and Di Marco, A.   FEBS Lett. (1972), 21, 264.
75. Chandra, P., Di Marco, A., Zunino, F., Casazza, A. M., Gericke, D., Giuliani, F., Soranzo, C., Thorbeck, R., Gotz, A., Arcamone, F., and Ghione, M.   Naturwiss. (1972), 59, 448.
76. Goodman, M. F., Bessman, M. J., and Bachur, N. R.   Proc. Nat. Acad. Sci. (1974), 71, 1193.
77. Di Marco, A., Casazza, A. M., Dasdia, T., Guiliani, F., Lenaz, L., Necco, A., and Soranzo, C.   Cancer Chemo. Rpts., Part 1 (1973), 57, 269.
78. Tobey, R. A.   Cancer Res. (1972), 32. 2720.
79. Kim, S. H. and Kim, J. H.   Cancer Res. (1972), 32, 323.
80. Kim, J. H., Gelbard, A. S., Djordjevic, B., King, S. H., and Perez, A. G.   Cancer Res. (1968), 28, 2437.
81. Bhuyan, B. K. and Fraser, T. J.   Cancer Chemo. Rpts., Part 1, (1974), 58, 149.
82. Silvestrini, R., Di Marco, A., and Dasdia, T.   Cancer Res. (1970), 30, 966.
83. Silvestrini, R., Di Marco, A., and Dasdia, T.   Riv. Istochim. Norm. Pathol. (1969), 14, 284.
84. Sandberg, J. S., Howsden, F. L., Di Marco, A., and Goldin, A.   Cancer Chemo. Rpts., Part 1 (1970), 54, 1.
85. Silvestrini, R., Gambarucci, C., and Dasdia, T.   Tumori (1970), 56, 137.

86. Razek, Aly, Valeriote, F., and Vietti, T. Cancer Res. (1972), 32, 1496.
87. Schwartz, H. S. and Grindey, G. B. Cancer Res. (1973), 33, 1837.
88. Casazza, A. M., Di Marco, A., and Di Cuonzo, G. Cancer Res. (1971), 31, 1971.
89. Schwartz, H. S. Cancer Chemo. Rpts., Part 1 (1974), 58, 55.
90. Schwartz, H. S. Res. Comm. Chem. Path. & Pharmacol. (1975), 10, 51.
91. Gosalvez, M., Blanco, M., Hunter, J., Miko, M., and Chance, B. Europ. J. Cancer (1974), 10, 567.
92. Iwamoto, Y., Hansen, I. L., Porter, T. H., and Folkers, K. Biochem. Biophys. Res. Comm. (1974), 58, 633.
93. Murphree, S. A., Hwang, K. M., and Sartorelli, A. C. Pharmacologist (1974), 16, 209. Abstr. Fall Meeting, Am. Soc. Pharmacol. & Exptl. Ther., Aug. 18-22, 1974, Montreal.
94. Hwang, K. M., Murphree, S. A., and Sartorelli, A. C. Cancer Res. (1974), 34, 3396.
95. Dano, Keld. Cancer Chemo. Rpts., Part 1 (1972), 56, 701.
96. Hasholt, Lis and Dano, Keld. Hereditas (1974), 77, 303.
97. Zunino, F. FEBS Lett. (1971), 18, 249.
98. Yamamoto, K., Acton, E. M., and Henry, D. W. J. Med. Chem. (1972), 15, 872.
99. Geran, R. I., Greenberg, N. H., MacDonald, M. M., Schumacher, A. M., and Abbott, B. J. Cancer Chemo. Rpts., Part 3 (1972), 3, 1.
100. Venditti, J. M., Johnson, R. K., Geran, R. I., and Abbott, B. J. Report of the Division of Cancer Treatment, NCI, Vol. 2, 1973, p. 2.199.
101. Maral, Rene, Ponsinet, Gerard, and Jolles, Georges. C. R. Acad. Sci. Paris (1972), 275, 301.
102. Jacquillat, C., Weil, M., Gemon, M. F., Izrael, V., Schaison, G., Boiron, M., and Bernard, J. Brit. Med. J., Nov. 25, 1972, p. 468.
103. Chauvergne, J. Nouvelle Press Med. (1973), No. 9, March 3, 1973.
104. Skovsgaard, Torben. Cancer Chemo. Rpts., Part 1 (1975), 59, 301.
105. Tong, George, Lee, W. W., Black, D. R., and Henry, D. W. J. Med. Chem. (1976), 19, in press.
106. Arcamone, F. et al. J. Med. Chem. (1974), 17, 335.
107. Lenaz, L., Necco, A., Dasdia, T., and Di Marco, A. Cancer Chemo. Rpts., Part 1 (1974), 58, 769.
108. Israel, M., Tinter, S. K., Lazarus, H., Brown, B., and Modest, E. J. Abstracts, Eleventh International Cancer Congress, Florence, Italy. October 1974, Vol. 4, pp. 752-753.
109. Israel, M., Modest, E. J., and Frei, Emil. Cancer Res. (1975), 35, 1365.

110. Tong, George and Henry, D. W.  In preparation.
111. Trouet, Andre, Deprez-de Campeneere, D., and de Duve, C.
     Nature New Biol. (1972), 239, 110.
112. Atassi, Ghanem, and Tagnon, H. J.  Europ. J. Cancer (1974),
     10, 399.
113. Trouet, A., Duprez-de Campeneere, D., de Smedt-Malengreaux,
     M., and Atassi, G.  Europ. J. Cancer (1974), 10, 405.
114. Sokal, G., Trouet, A., Michaux, J.-L., and Cornu, G.  Europ.
     J. Cancer (1973), 9, 391.
115. Cornu, G., Michaux, J.-L., Sokal, G., and Trouet, A.  Europ.
     J. Cancer (1974), 10, 695.
116. Marks, Thomas, Kline, Ira, and Venditti, J. M.  Proc. Am.
     Asso. Cancer Res. (1974), 16, 92.
117. Penco, S.  Chim. Ind., Milan (1968), 50, 908.
118. Di Marco, A., Zunino, F., Silvestrini, R., Gambarucci, C.,
     and Gambetta, R. A.  Biochem. Pharmacol. (1971), 20, 1323.
119. Arcamone, F., Penco, S., Vigevani, A., Redaelli, S.,
     Franchi, G., Di Marco, A., Casazza, A., Dasdia, T.,
     Formelli, F., Necco, A., and Soranzo, C.  J. Med. Chem.
     (1975), 18, 703.
120. Fujiwara, A. N., Wu, H., Lee, W. W., and Henry, D.  In
     preparation.
121. Lee, W. W., Wu, H. Y., Christensen, J. E., Goodman, Leon,
     and Henry, D. W.  J. Med. Chem. (1975), 18, 768..
122. Mosher, C. W. and Henry, D. W.  In preparation.
123. French Patent 1,593,555 (Rhone-Poulenc, July 10, 1970).
124. Fujiwara, A. N., Stankorb, J., Acton, E. M., Lee, W. W.,
     and Henry, D. W.  In preparation.
125. Lee, W. W., Martinez, A. P., and Henry, D. W.  Abstr. 167th
     Nat. Meeting of the Am. Chem. Soc., Los Angeles, April 1974.
     Abstr. No. MED1-58.
126. Muller, Werner, Flugel, Rolf, and Stein, Carl.  Liebigs
     Ann. Chim. (1971), 754, 15.
127. Double, J. C. and Brown, J. R.  J. Pharm. Pharmacol. (1975),
     27, 502.
128. Yamamoto, K., Acton, E. M., and Henry, D. W.  In prepara-
     tion.
129. Finkelstein, J. and Romano, J. A.  J. Med. Chem. (1970), 13,
     568.
130. Fujiwara, A. N., Acton, E. M., and Henry, D. W.  In prepara-
     tion.
131. Bicknell, R. B. and Henry, D. W.  In preparation.
132. Grange, E. W., Lee, W. W., and Henry, D. W.  In preparation.
133. Herman, E., Mhatre, R., Lee, I. P., Vick, J., and
     Waravdekar, V. S.  Pharmacology (1971), 6, 230.
134. Mhatre, R., Herman, E., Huidobro, A., and Waravdekar, V. J.
     Pharmacol Exptl. Therapeut. (1971), 178, 216.
135. Cargill, C., Bachmann, E., and Zbinden, G.  J. Nat. Cancer
     Inst. (1974), 53, 481.

136. Jaenke, R. S. Lab. Invest. (1974), 30, 292.
137. Young, D. M. and Fioravanti, J. L. Proc. Am. Asso. Cancer Res. (1974), 17, 73.
138. Necco, A. and Dasdia, T. IRCS Libr. Compend. (1974), 2, 1293.
139. Henry, D. W. Cancer Chemo. Rpts., Part 2 (1974), 4, 5.

# 3

# Biochemical Pharmacology of the Anthracycline Antibiotics

NICHOLAS R. BACHUR

Biochemistry Section, Baltimore Cancer Research Center, National Cancer Institute, 3100 Wyman Park Dr., Baltimore, Md. 21211

Medical scientists have a cumulative eighteen year clinical experience with the anthracycline antibiotics, adriamycin and daunorubicin. Daunorubicin was introduced into clinical trials in Italy by Farmitalia and in France by Rhône-Poulenc in 1964. A few years later, adriamycin was announced by Farmitalia and started into clinical trials. These trials indicated that daunorubicin was an impressive agent for remission induction in acute leukemia whereas adriamycin had a wider spectrum of activity against solid tumors as well as leukemias (1,2,3,4,5). There is little doubt that the anthracycline antibiotics isolated from Streptomyces have had a major impact on the prospects of cancer chemotherapy, because of their degree of activity for inducing remission or stopping progression of malignant growth and their wide ranging activity against malignancies. However, complicating their usefulness are the toxic side effects associated with their administration: myelosuppression, stomatitis, nausea, vomiting, alopecia, electrocardiographic changes, and a serious cumulative dosage related myocardiopathy (6).

Although the agents are nearly identical structurally (Fig. 1), adriamycin's potency is about one and one-half times greater than daunorubicin in both pharmacologic effect and in toxicity. The only difference between the complex molecules is at the number fourteen carbon position where adriamycin has an additional hydroxyl. Although many structures were reviewed extensively in the preceeding discussion by Dr. Henry, I think we can reexamine the fundamental structure from a biochemical view point. The antibiotic molecule is double headed with a hydrophobic end and a hydrophilic end. The A, B, and C resonating ring system comprises the hydrophobic end; and the D ring, with attached amino sugar are the hydrophilic head of the molecule. In addition to this dual physical characteristic, the molecules are amphoteric with a basic amino group and the acidic phenolic hydroxyls of the anthracycline ring. These physical properties plus abundance of reactive sites offer the potential for numerous interactions with cellular components such as nucleic acids, proteins, and lipids.

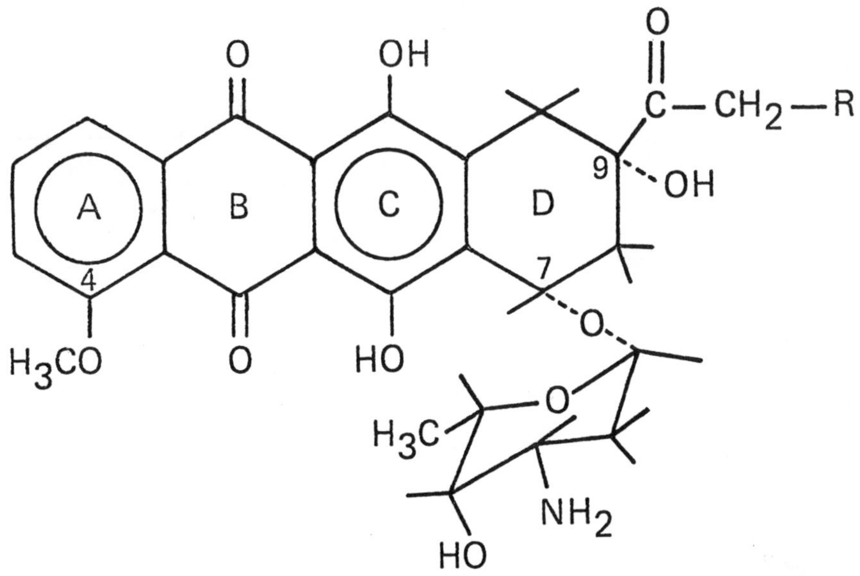

| | R |
|---|---|
| ADRIAMYCIN | OH |
| DAUNORUBICIN | H |

*Figure 1. Structures of adriamycin and daunorubicin*

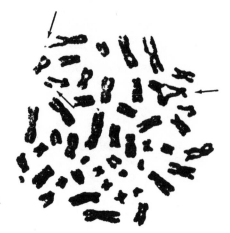

*Figure 2. Chromosomal damage in human cells induced by daunorubicin (10)*

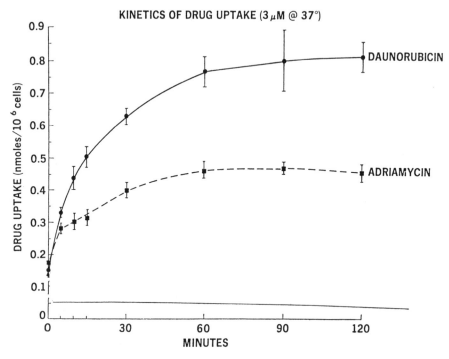

*Figure 3. Kinetics of adriamycin and daunorubicin uptake at 37°C in L1210 murine leukemia cells in vitro*

The availability of biotransformation groups increases even further the complications of drug disposition in mammals.

A central structural component of both molecules is the glycosidic bond joining the sugar, daunosamine, and the anthracycline nucleus. This bond is very labile to chemical and enzymatic cleavage; and the scission of the bond inactivates the compound. For this reason neither adriamycin nor daunorubicin are given orally since the glycosidic bond is split in the gastrointestinal tract. Both adriamycin and daunorubicin must be given parenterally to be effective.

When adriamycin or daunorubicin are administered intravenously to animals or in humans, the compounds are rapidly absorbed into cells and localized primarily in the cell nucleus (7,8,9). There is good anatomical and chemical evidence to indicate that the compounds both localize in the cell nucleus and also interact with the nuclear material. Chromosomal preparations from human lymphocytes show extensive damage after daunorubicin treatment (Fig. 2) (10). The chromosomes show fragmentation, ring formation, splitting, separation, and other forms of damage. Since both adriamycin and daunorubicin have a unique fluorescence, they can be detected by fluorescence microscopy in cells. With this technique the drug fluorescence is localized at the nuclear structures (8).

It is remarkable that the seemingly insignificant extra hydroxyl of adriamycin makes not only a more potent compound, but also a drug with wider spectrum of activity against malignancy. For this reason the drugs have been studied and compared. Since the whole animal studies are quite complex, we originally compared adriamycin and daunorubicin in mammalian cell culture containing L1210 murine leukemia cells. L1210 cells and other mammalian cell lines are inhibited more by daunorubicin than by adriamycin. Daunorubicin has a greater activity for inhibiting both DNA and RNA metabolism as seen in our laboratory and in others (Table 1) (11,12,13). This, of course, is the opposite of the clinical findings and of findings in vivo and was a perplexing observation. The possibility remained that the two drugs may be entering the cells at different rates, so we compared the accumulation of adriamycin and daunorubicin in the L1210 cells. Daunorubicin is taken into the cell much more rapidly and to a higher degree than is adriamycin (Fig. 3) (11). Therefore the effective level of drug in the cell is much higher in the case of daunorubicin. This results in an apparent superiority of daunorubicin over adriamycin at inhibiting nucleic acid synthesis. However, the specific activities of the amount of drug in the cells compared to the amount of inhibition produced by the drug indicates that adriamycin has a greater specific activity than does daunorubicin (11).

Alterations on the side chain at the 9 position have profound effects on the polarity and solubility of the anthracycline antibiotics. This apparently directly effects absorption of the drug

Table 1

In Vitro Inhibition of Cell Activities
by Adriamycin and Daunorubicin

| System | Adriamycin | Daunorubicin | Drug conc (μM) | Ref. |
|---|---|---|---|---|
| | Percent Inhibition | | | |
| 1. L1210 incorporation Thymidine-methyl $^3$H | 16<br>32<br>59 | 27<br>55<br>74 | 1<br>3<br>5 | Meriwether & Bachur (11) |
| 2. L1210 incorporation Uridine-2-$^{14}$C into RNA | 12<br>36<br>57 | 29<br>60<br>73 | 1<br>3<br>5 | Meriwether & Bachur (11) |
| | $ID_{50}$ μM | | | |
| 3. HeLa Cell survival | 1.9 | 0.9 | | DiMarco et al (12) |
| 4. HeLa Cell survival | 0.2 | 0.03 | | Kim & Kim (13) |

Table 2

Adriamycin and Daunorubicin Inhibition of DNA Polymerases

|  | Adr. | Daun. | Drug Conc. (mM) | Ref. |
|---|---|---|---|---|
|  | % Inhibition | | | |
| 1. E. Coli-T$_4$/L141 phage DNA polymerase | 22 | 15 | 0.011 | Goodman et al (14) |
|  | 58 | 39 | 0.028 | |
|  | 89 | 72 | 0.057 | |
|  | 98 | 95 | 0.114 | |
| 2. RNA Tumor Virus DNA Polymerase | | | | |
| Malony sarcoma virus | 67 | 67 | 0.066 | Chandra et al (15) |
| Friend Leukemia virus | 56 | 64 | 0.066 | |
| Rausher Sarcoma virus | 64 | 66 | 0.066 | |

into the cell. We have compared metabolites and chemical derivatives of adriamycin and daunorubicin with changes only on the C9
side chain. Compounds with the lowest "polarity" as measured by
partition coefficient have the highest uptake into L1210 cells.
There is a near linear relationship of polarity to drug uptake
(Fig. 4).

In order to avoid the dynamics of the cell membrane, we
investigated drug effects directly in vitro on a group of purified
DNA polymerases supplied by Dr. Maurice Bessman. The polymerases
were T4 bacteriophage induced in E. Coli. Inhibition of the DNA
polymerases was slightly greater with adriamycin than with daunorubicin (Table 2) (14). From our data and from the data of others
(Table 2) (15), it is difficult to explain why adriamycin has a
higher potency in mammals. The potency of the two agents is
nearly identical in these in vitro DNA polymerase assays. In
addition, their binding to DNA is quite similar and the unwinding
angle that they produce is very similar. This approach does not
explain the clinical differences seen with adriamycin and daunorubicin.

Studies on purified T4 phage induced polymerases uncovered
another unpredicted action of the anthracyclines which may have
significance in their selective action against malignant cells.
The purified phage polymerases fall into three phenotypic groups,
mutagenic, wild type, and antimutagenic. The mutagenic strains
have a high mutation frequency, the antimutagenic strains have a
low mutation frequency, and the wild type falls between with a
normal mutation rate. We observed that at low drug concentrations
the mutagenic polymerases were not inhibited but were stimulated
(ex., L56) (Fig. 5) whereas the antimutagenic polymerases (L141)
were uniformly inhibited as predicted (14). Simultaneously, a
5' exonuclease which is a part of each enzyme and is theorized to
be the editing or error correcting system for the phage DNA
synthesis is uniformly inhibited at all concentrations of the
drugs. This means that at low drug levels the mutagenic DNA
polymerase is made even more mutagenic since the low fidelity
polymerase is stimulated while the associated correction system
is inhibited. This does not occur in the antimutagenic enzymes
which are uniformly inhibited. This may be a clue to how these
drugs are selective for leukemic cells. Since the DNA polymerase
in acute leukemia cells is believed to be mutagenic (16), the
drugs may cause the leukemic cells to incorporate too many errors
into their DNA to be compatible with survival.

As previously stated, all of the studies investigating the
physical-chemical interactions of adriamycin and daunorubicin and
the comparative effects on cell and tissue culture inhibition, on
enzymes such as DNA polymerase and RNA polymerase, or on binding
to DNA have shown little if any difference between the two
compounds. It is only in whole animal studies that significant
differences between adriamycin and daunorubicin effects are easily
discernable. This indicates that other unrealized mechanisms are

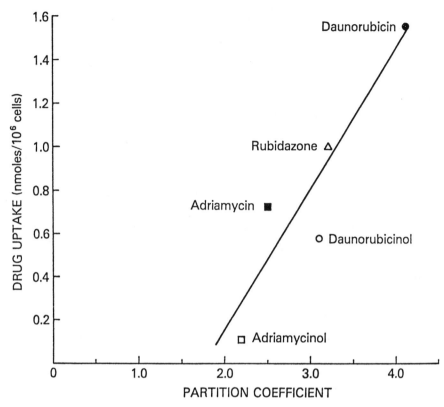

Figure 4.  *Relationship of drug uptake into L1210 cells and n-butanol–water partition coefficient of several anthracycline derivatives*

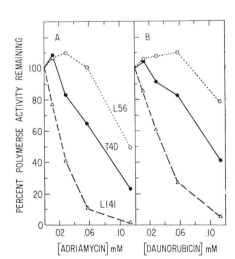

Figure 5.  *Effects of adriamycin and daunorubicin on DNA polymerases induced by T4 bacteriophage in* E. Coli (14)

responsible.  From that point of view we can examine other aspects
of the biochemical pharmacology of these compounds in the mammal
such as their metabolic disposition.  Patients treated with adriamycin or daunorubicin excrete significant quantities of the drugs
and the metabolites in the urine (17,18).  From these metabolites
we have been able to determine qualitatively and quantitatively
the metabolic sequences and pathways which the drugs traverse
(19).

The major metabolic step for both adriamycin and daunorubicin
in mammals is via the keto reduction reaction (20,21,22) (Fig. 6).
This reaction is catalyzed by a soluble aldo-keto reductase found
in all cells analyzed.  The enzyme requires NADPH as a cofactor
and produces the pharmacologically active products, daunorubicinol
and adriamycinol respectively from daunorubicin and adriamycin.
After animals are administered adriamycin, the parent drug is the
predominant material found in tissues at eight hours; but adriamycinol is a significant metabolite (22).  After daunorubicin
administration, daunorubicinol is the major drug form found in
tissues and excreted (22).  Since the aldo-keto reductase produces
pharmacologically active metabolites which differ from the parent
in physical-chemical characteristics, this enzyme and its level
in tumor and tissue may help determine the pharmacodynamic effects
of these drugs.  In studying the tissue distribution of aldo-keto
reductase, we examined human tissues obtained at autopsy.  All
human tissues examined contain active levels of aldo-keto
reductase (23).  Daunorubicin is a better substrate for the aldo-
keto reductases in most animal tissues and with purified aldo-keto
reductase preparations (21,22,23).

Both subsequent to or concurrent with carbonyl reduction, the
anthracycline glycosides are metabolized by glycosidases in most
tissues (20,24,25).  These microsomal enzymes split the drug or
reduced metabolites into aglycones and free amino sugar (Fig. 7)
(reactions:  I → IV, II → III, II → V).  The major glycosidase
(I → IV, II → V) is reductive in its mechanism, requires NADPH
for activity, produces deoxyaglycones (IV,V) and is inhibited by
oxygen (24).  As in the carbonyl reduction, daunorubicin is the
better substrate for the glycosidases than is adriamycin.  The
aglycone products of these reactions apparently have no anticancer
activity.  Since they are liberated intracellularly, however,
these aglycones may have activities which are not readily apparent
and more research is necessary to resolve this question.  The
aglycones because of their high lipid, low water solubility, are
excreted principally in the bile; but must be conjugated first to
increase water solubility (22,25,26,27,28).

Prior to conjugation, in order to offer a more appropriate
conjugation site, there is a 4-O demethylation of both daunorubicin and adriamycin to yield the demethylated aglycone (V → VI)
(19).  Demethylated aglycones serve as substrate for O-sulfation
and O-beta-glucuronidation yielding the 4-O-sulfate conjugate and
4-O-beta glucuronide conjugate (VI → VI, VI → VIII) to be

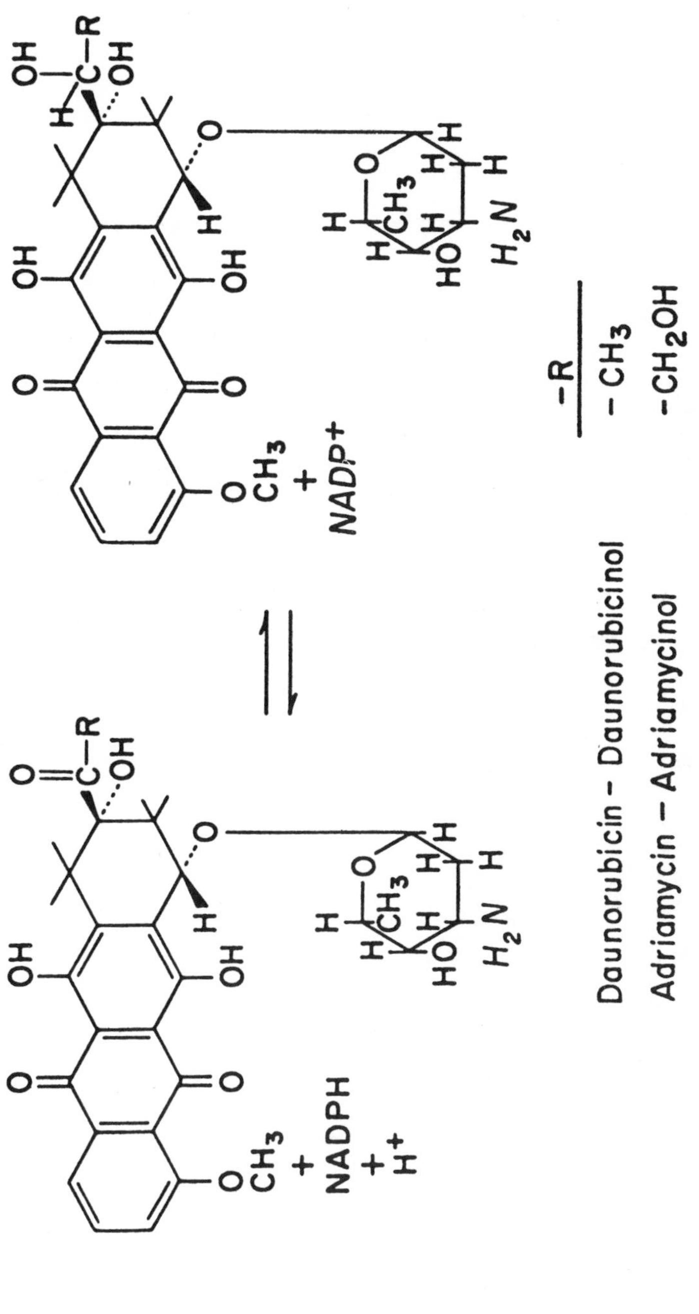

*Figure 6. Aldo-keto reductase reaction*

| | -R |
|---|---|
| Daunorubicin – Daunorubicinol | – CH₃ |
| Adriamycin – Adriamycinol | – CH₂OH |

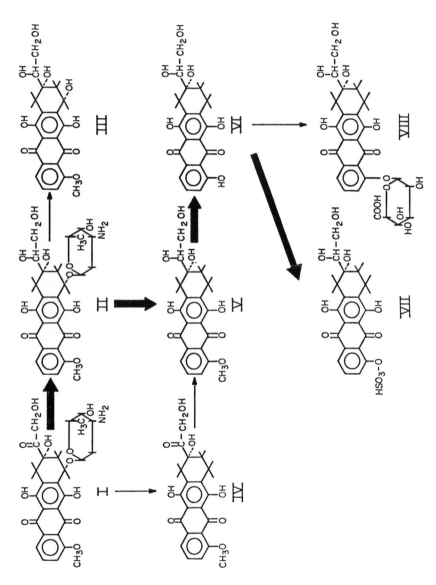

*Figure 7.    Pathways for human metabolism of adriamycin (19)*

excreted. All of these materials are found in human bile and human urine (26,27,28).

Since the reduced compounds, adriamycinol and daunorubicinol, show substantial anticancer activity, it is possible that other metabolites may have other types of activity. There are numerous metabolites with the potential for these substances to be biologically as well as pharmacologically active. The potentials are being examined at the present time.

Studies to date still have not explained fully the pharmacologic differences between adriamycin and daunorubicin. There are major differences in the disposition and metabolism of the agents in vivo and in the penetration through cell membranes as we have shown. Also differences in their effects on immunosuppression have been reported (29,30). The evidence is accumulating to define the precise mechanisms of action of these drugs.

The anthracycline antibiotics show promise as cancer chemotherapeutic agents. It is apparent that both adriamycin and daunorubicin have complex interactions with biologic systems. I feel that we can look forward to encouraging progress if we learn and understand more about the biological interactions of these agents. Then we may be better prepared to design analogs that are safer and more effective in their purpose.

LITERATURE CITED
1. Boiron, M., Jacquillat, C., Weil, M., Tanzer, J., Levy, D., Sultan, C., and Bernard, J.: Lancet (1969) 1, 330-333.
2. Wiernik, P.H. and Serpick, A.A.: Cancer Res. (1972) 32, 2023-2026.
3. Tan, C., Tasaka, H., Yu, K.P., Murphy, M.L., and Karnovsky, D. Cancer (1967) 20, 333.
4. Bonadonna, G., Monfardini, S., Delena, M., Fossati-Bellani, F. and Beretta, G.: Cancer Res. (1970) 30, 2572-2582.
5. Middleman, E., Luce, J., and Frei, E.: Cancer (1970) 28, 837-843.
6. Blum, R.H. and Carter, S.K.: Ann. Int. Med. (1974) 80, 249-259.
7. Bachur, N.R., Egorin, M.J., and Hildebrand, R.C.: Biochem. Med. (1973) 8, 352-361.
8. Egorin, M.J., Hildebrand, R.C., Cimino, E.F., and Bachur, N.R.: Cancer Res. (1974) 34, 2243-2245.
9. Silvestrini, R., Gambarucci, C., and Dasdia, T.: Tumori (1970) 56, 137-148.
10. Whang Peng, J., Leventhal, B.G., Adamson, J.W., and Perry, S. Cancer (1969) 23, 113-121.
11. Meriwether, W.D. and Bachur, N.R.: Cancer Res. (1972) 32, 1137-1142.
12. DiMarco, A., Zunino, F., Silvestrini, R., Gambarucci, C., and Gambetta, R.A.: Biochem. Pharmacol. (1971) 20, 1323-1328.

13. Kim, S.H. and Kim, J.H.: Cancer Res. (1972) 32, 323-325.
14. Goodman, M.F., Bessman, M.J., and Bachur, N.R.: Proc. Nat. Acad. Sci., USA (1974) 71, 1193-1196.
15. Chandra, P., Zunino, F., Gotz, D., Gericke, R., Thorbeck, R., and DiMarco, A.: FEBS Let. (1972) 21, 264-268.
16. Springgate, C.F. and Loeb, L.A.: Proc. Nat. Acad. Sci., USA (1973) 70, 245-249.
17. Huffman, D., Benjamin, R.S., and Bachur, N.R.: Clin. Pharmacol. Therap. (1972) 13, 895-905.
18. Benjamin, R.S., Riggs, C.E., Jr., and Bachur, N.R.: Clin. Pharmacol. Therap. (1973) 14, 592-600.
19. Takanashi, S. and Bachur, N.R.: Proc. Amer. Assoc. Cancer Res. (1974) 15, 76.
20. Bachur, N.R. and Gee, M.: J. Pharmacol. Exp. Ther. (1971) 177, 567-572.
21. Felsted, R.L., Gee, M., and Bachur, N.R.: J. Biol. Chem. (1974) 249, 3672-3679.
22. Bachur, N.R., Hildebrand, R.C., and Jaenke, R.S.: J. Pharmacol. Exp. Ther. (1974) 191, 331-340.
23. Bachur, N.R., Takanashi, S., Arena, E.: Proc. XI Inter. Cancer Congress, Florence, 1974.
24. Bachur, N.R. and Gee, M.: Fed. Proc. (1972) 31, 835.
25. Bullock, F.J., Bruni, R.J., and Asbell, A.: J. Pharmacol. Exp. Ther. (1972) 182, 70-76.
26. Cradock, J.C., Egorin, M.J., and Bachur, N.R.: Arch. Inter. Pharmacodyn. (1973) 202, 48-61.
27. Bachur, N.R., Egorin, M.J., Hildebrand, R.C., and Takanashi, S.: Proc. Amer. Assoc. Cancer Res. (1973) 14, 14.
28. Benjamin, R.S., Riggs, C.E., Jr., Serpick, A.A., and Bachur, N.R.: Clin. Res. (1974) 22, 483.
29. Schwartz, H.S. and Grindey, G.B.: Cancer Res. (1973) 33, 1837-1844.
30. Casazza, A.M.: Adriamycin 2nd Int. Sympos. Brussels, 1974.

# Potential Bioreductive Alkylating Agents

AI JENG LIN, LUCILLE A. COSBY, and ALAN C. SARTORELLI

Department of Pharmacology and Section of Developmental Therapeutics, Division of Oncology, Yale University School of Medicine, New Haven, Conn. 06510

Clinical tests of the past years have repeatedly demonstrated that alkylating agents represent one of the most effective therapies against various forms of cancer of man. These results encourage the expenditure of continuous effort to develop new types of alkylating agents with varied carrier groups designed to orient the alkylating portion of the molecule to different intracellular sites (1), as well as of derivatives which require unique modes of activation. Thus, alkylating agents, such as the nitrosoureas (2-4), cyclophosphamide (5,6), and the triazine derivatives (7-10), which require either enzymatic or chemical activation prior to alkylation, are examples of efficacious materials of this class with different neoplastic specificities. These alkylating agents may be classified as compounds with latent activity (11). The use of a latenization principle allows the design of compounds which may exploit biochemical differences between the most susceptible normal tissues and neoplastic cells. The effective employment of such a principle, ultimately, requires the biochemical monitoring of individual cancers to select those most prone to activate the latent alkylating potential.

Our interest in the development of potential bioreductive alkylating agents, a relatively new class of drugs which requires reductive activation prior to maximum exertion of alkylating potential, is based upon (a) the assumption that in the hypoxic neoplastic cells of solid tumors distal to blood vessels, which traditionally are extremely resistant to chemotherapy, the decreased oxygen tension creates conditions conducive to reduction; such cells should theoretically be particularly sensitive to quinones which require bioreduction prior to exertion of their growth-inhibitory potential, and (b) studies of the biochemical mechanism of action of mitomycin C, an antineoplastic agent which has activity against solid tumors of both animals and man (12-15). Thus, compounds of this type may be particularly useful against certain solid tumors.

Iyer and Szybalsky (16) have presented evidence to indicate that the mitomycins act as bifunctional alkylating agents which

71

add across both strands of the DNA double helix to cause cross-
linking. Furthermore, it has been demonstrated that (a) the reduction of the benzoquinone ring of the mitomycin molecule to
dihydrobenzoquinone was an essential step for biological activity
(17) and (b) an NADPH-dependent microsomal system was involved
in the reductive activation step (18,19). Kinoshita and his co-
workers (20,21) have reported a positive correlation between both
the antineoplastic and antimicrobial activities of a series of
mitomycin derivatives and their reduction potentials. These investigators have also provided evidence that the carbamyl group
and the aziridine ring of the mitomycins were not essential for
biological activity, proposing that the essential portions of the
mitomycin molecule were the structures shown in formulas I and
II (Scheme I). It is conceivable that charge delocalization
of the dihydroquinone hydroxyl groups of II results in o-quinone

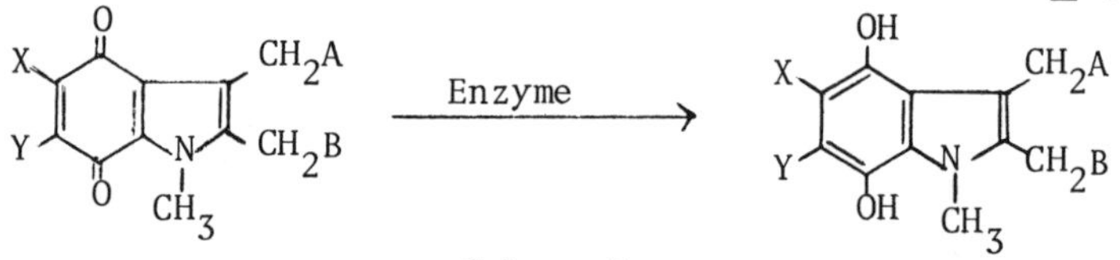

Scheme I

methide (III)-like intermediates, IV and V, which are the forms
that act to alkylate DNA (Scheme II).

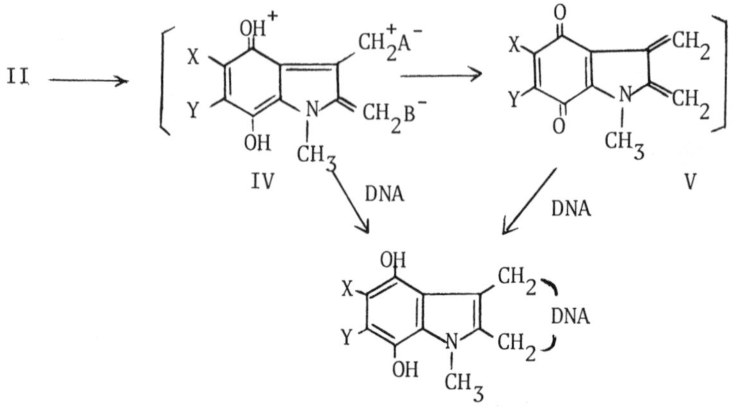

Scheme II

    o-Quinone methides (III) have been reported to be active
intermediates in several chemical reactions; indications for
their possible involvement in a number of biochemical processes
have also been published (22). In view of the similarities in
structure and in possible chemical reactivity between the pre-
sumed active form of the mitomycin analogs (V) and quinone

III                    VII                   VIII

methides (III), it was anticipated that bis(o-quinone methides)
(VII), generated in cells, would have the potential to alkylate
DNA, as well as other macromolecules of biological importance,
and thereby perhaps be effective tumor-inhibitory agents. Based
upon this concept, a series of benzo- and naphthoquinones (VIII),
possessing one or two side chains with the potential to alkylate
following reduction, were prepared (23-25).

Since the NADPH-dependent enzyme system which reduces the
mitomycins in vivo apparently has little specificity, conceivably
the same quinone reductase system will convert the quinones of
the bioreductive alkylating series to their corresponding dihydro-
quinones, a reaction essential for the expression of alkylating
potential. Furthermore, since Cater and Phillips (26) reported
a significantly lower oxidation-reduction potential for tumor
tissue, relative to most normal tissues, it is conceivable that
a therapeutic differential will exist between normal tissues
and some cancers for compounds requiring bioreductive activation.

## Antineoplastic Effects.

The naphthoquinone derivatives (Table I) of this series
produce significant prolongation of the life span of mice bearing
either Adenocarcinoma 755 or Sarcoma 180 ascites cells, with considerably greater potency being exhibited in the Adenocarcinoma
755 test system (24). Benzoquinone derivatives, however, were,
in general, only active against Adenocarcinoma 755 (23); an exception was 2,3-dimethyl-5,6-bis(chloromethyl)-1,4-benzoquinone,
which was also moderately active against Sarcoma 180. Among
the naphthoquinones tested (Table I), differences in maximal
activity between compounds in a given tumor system were relatively
small. Derivatives with two groups capable of alkylation after
bioreduction appeared to be equal in antitumor activity to agents
possessing only one arm with alkylating potential. Furthermore,
similarities were observed in the antineoplastic potencies of
chloromethyl, bromomethyl, and acetoxymethyl derivatives of
naphthoquinones, implying that the type of leaving group present
in the molecule was not critical for tumor inhibitory potency.

The mechanism of action of this class of compounds (Scheme
III) has been hypothesized (23,27) to involve bioreduction in
vivo, in a manner analogous to mitomycin C, presumably by an
NADPH-dependent quinone reductase enzyme system, although other

Table I. Antineoplastic Activities of Benzo- and Naphthoquinone Derivatives Against Sarcoma 180 and Adenocarcinoma 755 Ascites Cells.[a]

| Inhibitor | $R_1$ | $R_2$ | Adenocarcinoma 755[b] | Sarcoma 180[b] |
|---|---|---|---|---|
| None | -- | -- | 13.3 | 11.8 |
| | $-CH_2Cl$ | $-H$ | 47.6 | 23.4 |
| | $-CH_2Cl$ | $-CH_3$ | 39.8 | 19.2 |
| | $-CH_2Cl$ | $-CH_2Cl$ | 38.6 | 22.6 |
| | $-CH_2Br$ | $-CH_3$ | 45.4 | 25.0 |
| | $-CH_2Br$ | $-H$ | 47.6 | 24.6 |
| | $-CH_2OAc$ | $-H$ | 29.8 | 16.8 |
| | $-CH_2OAc$ | $-CH_2OAc$ | -- | 22.8 |
| | $-CH_3$ | $-H$ | -- | 10.4 |
| | $-CH_2Cl$ | $-CH_2Cl$ | -- | 18.5 |
| | $-CH_2OAc$ | $-CH_2OAc$ | 28.7 | 14.0 |
| | $-CH_2OAc$ | $-H$ | 37.0 | 12.4 |
| | $-CH_2OAc$ | $-H$ | -- | 9.4 |
| | $-CH_2OAc$ | $-H$ | 39.8 | 11.2 |

[a]Administered once daily for 6 consecutive days, beginning 24 hr after tumor implantation.
[b]Average survival time (days) of tumor-bearing mice at the optimal dosage schedule.

possibilities cannot be discounted, to form corresponding dihydro-quinones (X). The dihydroquinones are unstable and spontaneously decompose to form the anticipated reactive intermediates, o-quinone methides (VII). Such reactive species presumably then function as inhibitors of neoplastic growth by alkylation of DNA, RNA, and/or other biological materials in a manner similar to that of the mitomycins.

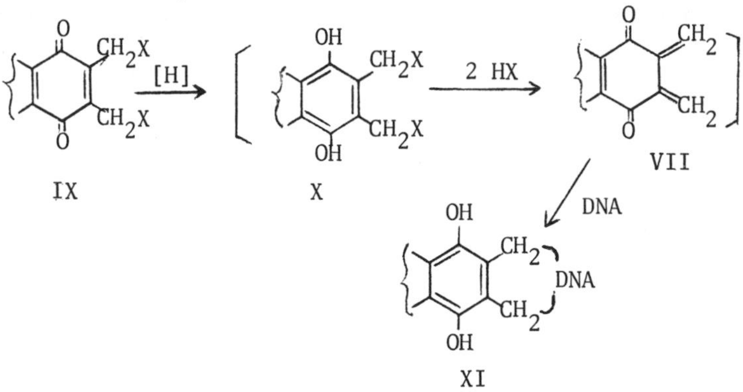

Scheme III

Although no biochemical evidence is currently available to support the existence of an o-quinone methide *in vivo*, chemical evidence (28) has been obtained to substantiate the formation

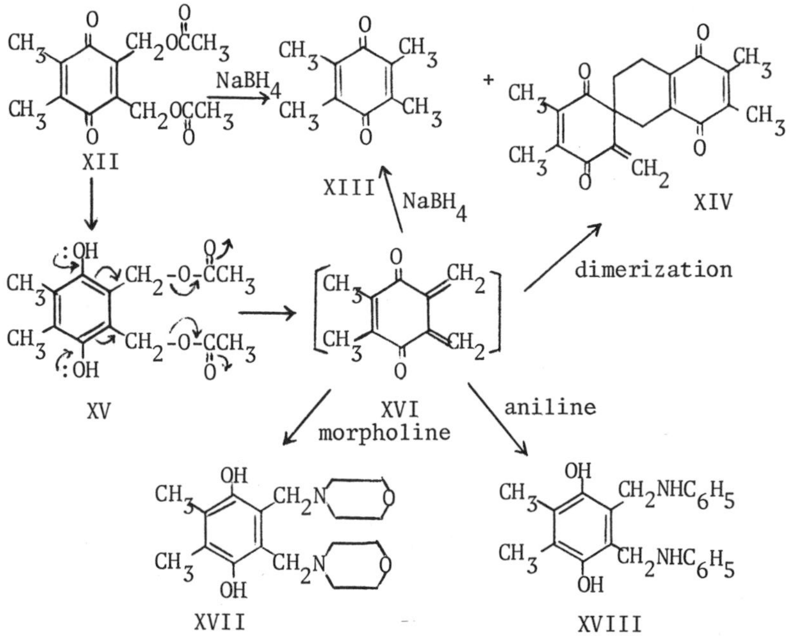

Scheme IV

of this intermediate in the reductive amination of 2,3-dimethyl-5,6-bis(acetoxymethyl)-1,4-benzoquinone (XII) by aniline and morpholine. This was demonstrated by reducing compound XII with 1 molar equivalent of NaBH$_4$ in methanol at ice-cold temperature (Scheme IV). Two major yellow products were obtained after column chromatography on silica gel. These products were identified as duroquinone (XIII) and the spiro dimer, 3',4'-dihydro-3,4,6',7'-tetramethyl-6-methylenespiro[3-cyclohexene-1,2'(1'H)-naphthalene]-2,5,5',8'-tetradone (XIV). The mechanism involved in the formation of products XIII and XIV can best be explained by the initial reduction of compound XII by NaBH$_4$ to the corresponding dihydro-benzoquinone XV, which decomposes to generate XVI. Further reduction or dimerization of XVI produces the observed products XIII and XIV. To provide additional evidence for the existence of XVI, the reduction of XII by NaBH$_4$ was carried out in the presence of morpholine and aniline. The expected adducts XVII and XVIII were obtained in high yield. The capability of intermediate XVI to alkylate aniline or morpholine suggested a similar potential to covalently bind to biological materials in vivo, if intermediate XVI were generated enzymatically in vivo.

The concept of bioreductive activation of these quinones requires strict structural constraints which allow the generation of an o-quinone methide, as well as a redox potential for the quinone ring that is compatible with biological activation. Studies of the relationships between structure and activity with a series of benzo- and naphthoquinone derivatives of this class have demonstrated that essentially all compounds possessing the quinone ring and an appropriate side chain(s) have antitumor activity (23,24); whereas, compounds with a side chain(s) ultimately capable of alkylation, but without the quinone nucleus or vice versa (Table II), were totally devoid of antineoplastic potency. These findings were interpreted to indicate that these molecules were unable to generate the required o-quinone methide intermediate.

Table II.   Some Compounds Devoid of Antineoplastic Activity
            Against Sarcoma 180 Which Demonstrate Structural
            Requirements for Bioreductive Alkylating Agents

2,5-Dimethoxy-3,4-dimethyl-1-chloromethylbenzene

2,5-Dimethoxy-3,4-dimethyl-1-acetoxymethylbenzene

2,5-Dimethoxy-3,4-dimethyl-1,2-bis(acetoxymethyl)benzene

2-Methyl-1,4-naphthoquinone

2-Acetoxyethyl-1,4-naphthoquinone

2,3,5,6-Tetramethyl-1,4-benzoquinone (duroquinone)

4. LIN ET AL. *Bioreductive Alkylating Agents* 77

Preliminary studies (29), on the relationship between the half-wave potentials (E1/2) of a series of benzo- and naphthoquinone derivatives of this class and their antitumor effects, indicated that compounds with relatively low redox potentials generally possessed the most efficacious antitumor activities, with the exception of 2,3-dimethyl-5,6-bis(chloromethyl)-1,4-benzoquinone which has moderate antitumor activity, even though its redox potential was in the range of Sarcoma 180 inactive materials (Table III). If the correlation between redox

Table III. Half-Wave Potential ($E_{1/2}$) and Antineoplastic Activity Against Sarcoma 180 of Benzo- and Naphthoquinones

| Inhibitor | $R_1$ | $R_2$ | Antineoplastic Activity | $E_{1/2}$ (volt) |
|---|---|---|---|---|
| (naphthoquinone structure with $R_1$, $R_2$) | $-CH_2Cl$ | $-CH_2Cl$ | + | -0.23 |
| | $-CH_2Cl$ | $-CH_3$ | + | -0.24 |
| | $-CH_2Cl$ | $-H$ | + | -0.24 |
| | $-CH_2Br$ | $-CH_2Br$ | + | -0.21 |
| | $-CH_2OAc$ | $-CH_2OAc$ | + | -0.21 |
| (2,3-dimethyl benzoquinone structure with $R_1$, $R_2$) | $-CH_2Cl$ | $-CH_2Cl$ | + | -0.05 |
| | $-CH_2OAc$ | $-CH_2OAc$ | - | -0.11 |
| | $-CH_2OAc$ | $-H$ | - | -0.11 |
| (2,3-dimethoxy benzoquinone structure with $R_1$, $R_2$) | $-CH_2OAc$ | $-CH_2OAc$ | - | -0.05 |
| | $-CH_2OAc$ | $-H$ | - | -0.06 |

potential and antitumor activity is an important feature for compounds of this class, it would be expected that materials with even lower redox potentials might exhibit more potent antineoplastic properties. In an effort to alter the redox potential significantly, an electron donating (methyl) and an electron withdrawing (chloro) group were introduced into the benzenoid ring of 2,3-bis(chloromethyl)-1,4-naphthoquinone. The results obtained (Table IV) indicate that the introduction of a methyl- or chlorofunction into the 5- or 6- position of the parent compound does not significantly affect either the redox potential or the antitumor activity of the parent compound. A similar observation,

Table IV. Half-Wave Potential ($E_{1/2}$) and Antineoplastic Activity
Against Sarcoma 180 of Some 5- or 6-Substituted
Naphthoquinones[a]

| $R_1$ | $R_2$ | $E_{1/2}$ (volt) | Av. survival time (days)[b] |
|---|---|---|---|
| Control | | | 12.4 |
| Cl | H | -0.26 | 25.0 |
| H | Cl | -0.28 | 21.8 |
| CH$_3$ | H | -0.28 | 25.8 |
| H | CH$_3$ | -0.31 | 19.4 |

[a]Administered once daily for 6 consecutive days, beginning 24 hr
after tumor implantation.
[b]Average survival time of tumor-bearing mice at the optimal dosage
schedule.

that substituents on the benzenoid ring of the naphthoquinone nucleus have little effect on the redox potential of the quinonoid
ring, has been reported (30). Furthermore, it has been shown that
substituents on the quinonoid ring of the naphthoquinone moiety
exert stronger effects on the redox potential of the ring than
substituents on the benzenoid ring (30). In addition, earlier
studies on the relationship between structure and activity in a
series of naphthoquinone derivatives of this class indicated that
compounds with one side chain capable of alkylation following reduction are as active as agents with two alkylating side chains
(23,24). Based upon these considerations, another series of 2-
chloromethyl- and 2-bromomethyl-1,4-naphthoquinone derivatives
with various substituents at the 3-position was prepared and their
redox potentials and antitumor effects against Sarcoma 180 were
measured (Table V) (31). These derivatives were found to be relatively potent inhibitors of the growth of Sarcoma 180 ascites
cells, with the exception of 2-chloromethyl-3-benzamido-1,4-
naphthoquinone, which was inactive against this tumor cell line.

Table V. Half-Wave Potential ($E_{1/2}$) and Antitumor Effects Against Sarcoma 180 of 2-Halomethyl-1,4-Naphthoquinones[a]

| R | X | $E_{1/2}$ (volt) | Av. survival time (days)[b] |
|---|---|---|---|
| $C_6H_5$ | Cl | -0.28 | 29.7 |
| $NHCC_6H_5$ (O) | Cl | -0.23 | 13.0 |
| $SC_2H_5$ | Cl | -0.27 | 30.4 |
| $SC_6H_5$ | Cl | -0.23 | 23.2 |
| Br | Br | -0.24 | 29.8 |
| Cl | Br | -0.25 | 29.8 |
| Mitomycin C | | -0.44 | 40.9 |
| Control | | | 12.4 |

[a]Administered once daily for 6 consecutive days, beginning 24 hr after tumor implantation.
[b]Average survival of tumor-bearing mice at the optimal dosage schedule.

Although the optimal daily dosage level of 15 mg/kg of 3-phenyl-2-chloromethyl-1,4-naphthoquinone was about equal in maximal activity to that of 3-chloro- or 3-bromo-2-bromomethylnaphthoquinone, the 3-phenyl derivative produced satisfactory antitumor activity over a wider range of dose levels, suggesting that this agent had the highest therapeutic index. However, the redox potentials and the antitumor effects of these compounds were found to be similar to those of the parent compound, indicating that the functional groups introduced into the molecule had minimal effect on the redox potential of the quinonoid ring, corresponding to the relatively minor effects of these materials on antitumor activity relative to the parent compound. Although hydroxyl and amino functions were reported to decrease the redox potential when introduced onto the quinonoid ring of the naphthoquinones (30), substitution of these functional groups onto the 3-position of 2-chloromethyl-1,4-naphthoquinone would be expected to result in an unstable molecule due to an electronic effect.

Table VI.  Antineoplastic Activity Against Sarcoma 180 of Quino-
line-5,8-dione and Naphthazarin Derivatives[a]

| Inhibitor | Av. survival time (days)[b] |
|---|---|
| None | 12.4 |
| | 18.6 |
| | 19.6 |
| | 19.6 |
| | 11.2 |
| | 14.4 |
| | 10.4 |

[a]Administered once daily for 6 consecutive days, beginning 24 hr
after tumor implantation.
[b]Average survival time of tumor-bearing mice at the optimal
dosage schedule.

It is interesting to note that the half-wave potential for
mitomycin C under the same experimental conditions was found to
be -0.44 volts, a value considerably lower than any of the compounds of this series; furthermore, its antitumor activity in this
system was also considerably greater. These results encourage the
further design and synthesis of compounds of the bioreductive
alkylating type with redox potentials lower than those already
available.

Both benzo- and naphthoquinone derivatives of this series
generally are poorly water soluble. This factor adds to the com-
plication of the ultimate preparation of a suitable parenteral
dosage form. As part of a study to develop new antineoplastic
agents of this class with (a) lower redox potentials and thus
possibly greater therapeutic potency, and (b) better water solubility (in salt form), the synthesis of a number of 2-chloro-
methyl- and 2-bromomethyl derivatives of naphthazarins and 2,3-
bis(bromomethyl)quinoline-5,8-dione was carried out (31). These
compounds (Table VI) were found to possess moderate antitumor activity, prolonging the life span of tumor-bearing mice from 12 to
13 days for untreated tumor-bearing control animals to 19 to 20
days. However, these results were obtained at the expense of substantial host toxicity, as measured by body weight loss during the
drug treatments. 2-Bromomethyl-3-bromo-6,7-dimethylnaphthazarin
was found to be inactive against Sarcoma 180 at dosage levels up
to 40 mg/kg per day, and as expected, 6,7-dimethylquinoline-5,8-
dione and 2,3-dibromo-1,2,3,4-tetrahydro-5,8-dimethoxy-2,3-
methylene-1,4-dioxonaphthalene, precursors of the final product,
were found to be inactive as antineoplastic agents. These results
further substantiated the validity of the proposed model compound
(VIII).

Biochemical Studies.

The involvement of coenzyme Q (CoQ) in mitochondrial electron
transport has been well recognized in biological systems. Mammalian succinoxidase and NADH-oxidase systems have been extensively
studied and may be considered representative of CoQ electron
transport sequences. A relationship has been documented between
antimalarial potency of benzoquinone and naphthoquinone derivatives and the degree of inhibition of mitochondrial succinoxidase
activity (32-34), a finding indicative of the importance of CoQ
to this parasite (35); however, no comparable evidence is available to indicate a similar relationship between antineoplastic
activity of quinone derivatives and inhibition of electron transport. Profound effects of ethyleneiminoquinones, which are relatively potent antineoplastic agents, on the respiration of carcinoma cells have been reported earlier (36,37).

These considerations prompted an investigation of the effects
of the bioreductive alkylating agents synthesized in this laboratory on beef heart mitochondrial NADH-oxidase and succinoxidase

Table VII.  Inhibition of Mitochondrial Succinoxidase and NADH-oxidase by Naphthoquinone Derivatives

| R1 | R2 | NADH-oxidase, %a | | | Succinoxidase, %a | | |
|---|---|---|---|---|---|---|---|
| | | $3.3 \times 10^{-4}$Mb | $1.7 \times 10^{-4}$Mb | $3.3 \times 10^{-5}$Mb | $3.3 \times 10^{-4}$Mb | $1.7 \times 10^{-4}$Mb | $3.3 \times 10^{-5}$Mb |
| CH2Cl | CH2Cl | 36.2+8.6 | | 60.3+7.2 | 10.9+6.1 | | 95.4+9.7 |
| CH2Cl | CH3 | 51.5+9.9 | | 51.7+14.7 | 16.8+7.7 | | 70.8+19.0 |
| CH2Cl | H | 47.1+7.7 | | 87.6+12.7 | 24.1+9.8 | | 95.4+5.2 |
| CH2Br | CH2Br | | 23.7+3.8 | 53.4+16.3 | | 16.0+3.8 | 55.3+23.4 |
| CH2Br | CH3 | | 29.2+3.3 | 46.1+11.6 | | 24.8+5.0 | 73.2+8.7 |
| CH2Br | H | | 20.0+4.3 | 81.7+19.8 | | 20.2+3.1 | 24.1+3.8 |
| CH2OC(O)CH3 | CH2OC(O)CH3 | 23.6+8.5 | | 74.5+19.1 | 24.5+5.8 | | 96.3+17.6 |
| CH2OC(O)CH3 | CH3 | 42.9+5.0 | | 37.4+7.1 | 71.3+10.9 | | 91.2+4.6 |
| CH2OC(O)CH3 | H | 31.0+4.4 | | 69.5+15.3 | 4.3+5.2 | | 95.6+5.4 |

aPer cent of uninhibited controls + standard deviation.  bConcentration of inhibitor employed.
[From: J. Med. Chem., 16, 1268, 1973; courtesy of the American Chemical Society].

activities. The results (Table VII) indicated that at concentrations of 1.7 to 3.3 x $10^{-4}$M, all quinones tested depressed mitochondrial succinoxidase and NADH-oxidase activities to about 50% or less of the uninhibited controls, except for 2-methyl-3-acetoxymethylnaphthoquinone. At a lower concentration (3.3 x $10^{-5}$M), only bromomethylnaphthoquinone ($R_1$ = -CH$_2$Br; $R_2$ = H) strongly inhibited succinoxidase activity (i.e., to below 30% of the uninhibited control). Interestingly, at the same concentration (3.3 x $10^{-5}$M), bromomethylnaphthoquinone only weakly decreased NADH-oxidase activity. This finding suggests a site of action by this compound at Complex II (i.e., succinate-CoQ reductase). In contrast, the three compounds with a 2-methyl group ($R_2$ = CH$_3$) tested, selectively inhibited NADH-oxidase activity at 3.3 x $10^{-5}$M, to at least 50% of control activity. This suggests a preferential site of action at Complex I (i.e., NADH-CoQ reductase). Among these three methyl compounds, the chloromethyl ($R_1$ = CH$_2$Cl; $R_2$ = CH$_3$) and acetoxymethyl ($R_1$ = CH$_2$OAc; $R_2$ = CH$_3$) analogs showed an equal degree of inhibition of NADH-oxidase activity at the two concentrations tested. Introduction of a lipoidal side chain (pentadecyl) into the acetoxymethyl or chloromethylbenzoquinone or naphthoquinone analogs resulted in a reduction of enzyme inhibitory activity (Table VIII) and complete elimination of antitumor activity (38). These results suggest that the lipoidal side chain may cause steric interference with the reactive alkylating side chain of the inhibitor molecule or that lipophilicity plays a negative role in the biological action of these compounds. The greater potency of the benzoquinones relative to naphthoquinones as inhibitors of CoQ-mediated enzyme systems does not correspond to their lesser activities when compared to naphthoquinone derivatives as antineoplastic agents, suggesting that the susceptibility of mitochondrial electron transport is not the major or sole determinant in the biochemical mechanism of action of this class of compounds. Accordingly, other potential metabolic sites of action have been sought. 2,3-Bis(chloromethyl)-1,4-naphthoquinone, a member of this series which is a relatively potent inhibitor of the growth of both Adenocarcinoma 755 and Sarcoma 180, has been found to cause greater inhibition of the synthesis of DNA in vivo than of the formation of either RNA or protein (39). For example, a single dose of 30 mg/kg of this compound produced 80% inhibition of the incorporation of thymidine-H$^3$ into DNA, with inhibition persisting for up to 24 hours after drug treatment. Radioactivity from C$^{14}$-labeled 2,3-bis(chloromethyl)-1,4-naphthoquinone was found to bind tightly to DNA, RNA, and protein isolated from Sarcoma 180 ascites cells exposed to this agent, suggesting the possible alkylation of these cellular macromolecules. This compound also changed the sedimentation pattern in alkaline sucrose gradients of DNA from drug-treated cells, indicating introduction of single strand breaks in these molecules.

Table VIII.  Inhibition of Beef Heart Mitochondrial NADH-Oxidase and Succinoxidase by Some Benzoquinone and Naphthoquinone Bioreductive Alkylating Agents

| $R_1$ | $R_2$ | NADH-oxidase (% control act.)[a] | | Succinoxidase (% control act.)[a] | |
|---|---|---|---|---|---|
| | | $3.3 \times 10^{-4}$ M[b] | $3.3 \times 10^{-5}$ M[b] | $3.3 \times 10^{-4}$ M[b] | $3.3 \times 10^{-5}$ M[b] |
| $-CH_3$ | $-H$ | 34.7 ± 5.2 | 39.2 ± 15.6 | 9.1 ± 0.8 | 39.3 ± 18.1 |
| $-OCH_3$ | $-H$ | 39.7 ± 17.2 | 103.9 ± 21.1 | 13.8 ± 3.6 | 63.5 ± 26.4 |
| $-CH_3$ | $-(CH_2)_{14}CH_3$ | 22.4 ± 14.4 | 93.9 ± 24.1 | 54.9 ± 8.6 | 89.2 ± 14.9 |
| $-OCH_3$ | $-(CH_2)_{14}CH_3$ | 17.4 ± 0.4 | 89.9 ± 3.6 | 50.3 ± 5.6 | 91.9 ± 8.0 |

| X | $R_1$ | NADH-oxidase (% control act.)[a] | | Succinoxidase (% control act.)[a] | |
|---|---|---|---|---|---|
| | | $3.3 \times 10^{-4}$ M[b] | $3.3 \times 10^{-5}$ M[b] | $3.3 \times 10^{-4}$ M[b] | $3.3 \times 10^{-5}$ M[b] |
| $-O_2CCH_3$ | $-H$ | 31.0 ± 4.4 | 69.5 ± 15.3 | 4.3 ± 5.2 | 95.6 ± 5.4 |
| $-Cl$ | $-H$ | 47.4 ± 7.7 | 87.6 ± 12.7 | 24.1 ± 9.8 | 95.4 ± 5.2 |
| $-O_2CCH_3$ | $-(CH_2)_{14}CH_3$ | 35.0 ± 3.9 | 80.2 ± 17.6 | 44.2 ± 8.8 | 89.9 ± 9.7 |
| $-Cl$ | $-(CH_2)_{14}CH_3$ | 91.9 ± 4.1 | 113.8 ± 13.3 | 86.6 ± 2.4 | 104.4 ± 7.3 |

[a] Percent of uninhibited controls ± standard deviation.
[b] Concenration of inhibitor employed. [From: J. Med. Chem. 17, 668, 1974; courtesy of the American Chemical Society.]

The biochemical data available to date indicate that this class of agents produces a variety of metabolic lesions in susceptible neoplastic cells, a finding presumably indicative of their alkylating potential.

## Literature Cited

1. Schnitzer, R. J., and Hawking, F., Experimental Chemother., Volume V, pp. 1-94, Academic Press, New York, 1967.
2. Johnston, T.P., McCaleb, G. S., and Montgomery, J. A., J. Med. Chem., (1963) 6, 669-681.
3. Schabel, F. M., Jr., Johnston, T. P., McCaleb, G. S., Montgomery, J. A., Laster, W. R., and Skipper, H. E., Cancer Res., (1963) 23, 725-733.
4. Nies, B. A., Thomas, L. B., and Freireich, E. J., Cancer, (1965) 18, 546-553.
5. Arnold, H., Bourseaux, F., and Brock, N., Naturwissensch., (1958) 45, 64-66.
6. Arnold, H., Bourseaux, F., and Brock, N., Nature (London) (1958) 181, 931.
7. Shealy, Y. F., Montgomery, J. A., and Laster, W. R., Jr., Biochem. Pharmacol., (1962) 11, 674-675.
8. Gerulath, A. H., and Loo, T. L., Biochem. Pharmacol., (1972) 21, 2335-2343.
9. Luce, J. K., Thurman, W. R., Isaacs, B. L., and Talley, R. W., Cancer Chemother. Rep., (1970) 54, 119-124.
10. Kingra, G. S., Comis, R., Olson, K. B., and Horton, J., Cancer Chemother. Rep., (1971) 55, 281-283.
11. Ross, W. C. J., Biological Alkylating Agents, pp. 177-180, Butterworths, London, 1962.
12. Livingston, R. B., and Carter, S. K., Single Agents in Cancer Chemotherapy, pp. 385-388, IFI/Plenum, New York, 1970.
13. Frank, W., and Osterberg, A. E., Cancer Chemother. Rep., (1960) 9, 114-119.
14. Sugiura, K., Cancer Res., (1959) 19, 438-445.
15. Miller, E., Sullivan, R. D., and Chryssochoos, T., Cancer Chemother. Rep., (1962) 21, 129-135.
16. Iyer, V. N., and Szybalski, W., Proc. Nat. Acad. Sci. U.S., (1963) 50, 355-362.
17. Schwartz, H. S., Sodergren, J. E., and Philips, F. S., Science, (1963) 142, 1181-1183.
18. Schwartz, H. S., J. Pharmacol. Exp. Ther., (1962) 136, 250-258.
19. Iyer, V. N., and Szybalski, W., Science (1964), 145, 55-58.
20. Kinoshita, S., Uzu, K., Nakano, K., Shimizu, M., Takahashi, T., and Matsui, M., J. Med. Chem., (1971) 14, 103-109.
21. Kinoshita, S., Uzu, K., Nakano, K., and Takahashi, T., J. Med. Chem., (1971) 14, 109-112.
22. Turner, A. B., Quart. Rev. Chem. Soc., (1964) 18, 347-360.

23. Lin, A. J., Cosby, L. A., Shansky, C. W., and Sartorelli, A. C., J. Med. Chem. (1972) 15, 1247-1252.
24. Lin, A. J., Pardini, R. S., Cosby, L. A., and Sartorelli, A. C., J. Med. Chem., (1973) 16, 1268-1271.
25. Lin, A. J., Shansky, C. W., and Sartorelli, A. C., J. Med. Chem., (1974) 17, 558-561.
26. Cater, D. B., and Phillips, A. F., Nature (London), (1954) 174, 121-123.
27. Lin, A. J., Cosby, L. A., and Sartorelli, A. C., Cancer Chemother. Rep., (1974) 4, 23-25.
28. Lin, A. J., and Sartorelli, A. C., J. Org. Chem., (1973) 38, 813-815.
29. Lin, A. J., and Sartorelli, A. C., Biochem. Pharmacol., (1975), in press.
30. Fieser, L. F., and Fieser, M., J. Amer. Chem. Soc., (1935) 57, 491-494.
31. Lin, A. J., Lillis, B. J., and Sartorelli, A. C., J. Med. Chem., (1975), in press.
32. Schnell, J. V., Siddiqui, W. A., Geiman, Q. M., Skelton, F. S., Lunan, K. D., and Folkers, K., J. Med. Chem., (1971) 14, 1026-1029.
33. Skelton, F. S., Pardini, R. S., Heidker, J. C., and Folkers, K., J. Amer. Chem. Soc., (1968) 90, 5334-5336.
34. Catlin, J. C., Pardini, R. S., Daves, G. D., Jr., Heidker, J. C., and Folkers, K., J. Amer. Chem. Soc., (1968) 90, 3572-3574.
35. Skelton, F. S., Lunan, K. D., Folkers, K., Schnell, J. V., Siddiqui, W. A., and Geiman, Q. M., Biochemistry, (1969) 8, 1284-1287.
36. Hayashi, S., Ueki, H., and Ueki, Y., Gann (1963) 54, 381-390.
37. Hayashi, S., Ueki, H., and Ueki, Y., Gann (1964) 55, 1-8.
38. Lin, A. J., Pardini, R. S., Lillis, B. J., and Sartorelli, A. C., J. Med. Chem., (1974) 17, 668-672.
39. Cosby, L. A., Lin, A. J., and Sartorelli, A. C., unpublished data.

# A Review of Studies on the Mechanism of Action of Nitrosoureas

GLYNN P. WHEELER

Southern Research Institute, 2000 Ninth Ave. S., Birmingham, Ala. 35205

This review supplements and updates several previous reviews (1,2,3,4), and some of the material covered in those reviews will be included here to provide background for more recent developments and to present an overview of this subject. However, some of the details and literature references that were given previously will not be repeated.

## Historical Background

In 1959 the routine screening of compounds for therapeutic activity against murine leukemia L1210, under the auspices of the Cancer Chemotherapy National Service Center, showed that N-methyl-N'-nitro-N-nitrosoguanidine (MNNG) was somewhat active. This finding stimulated the initiation of an investigation of compounds that might be progenitors of diazomethane, with nitrosoguanidines being studied at Stanford Research Institute (5,6) and the nitrosoureas being studied at Southern Research Institute. It was soon found that replacement of the methyl group on the nitrosated nitrogen atom of each series of compounds by a 2-haloethyl group gave improved anticancer activity and also that the nitrosoureas were more active agents than the nitrosoguanidines.

An additional stimulus for pursuing the study of nitrosoureas at Southern Research Institute was the observation by Skipper, Schabel, Trader, and Thomson (7) that in contrast to methotrexate, 6-mercaptopurine, cyclophosphamide, azaserine, 5-fluorouracil, mitomycin C, and MNNG, intraperitoneally administered N-methyl-N-nitrosourea (MNU) was active against intracerebrally inoculated L1210 cells. In the continuing program of preparation and evaluation of nitrosoureas by Johnston, McCaleb, Montgomery, and collaborators, early results (8) showed that N,N'-disubstituted-N-nitrosoureas were active compounds.  Subsequent tests (**9**,**10**) led to the conclusion that greater activity was obtained when the substituent on N-1 was a 2-chloroethyl or a 2-fluoroethyl group and the substituent on N-3 was a 2-chloroethyl, 2-fluoroethyl, cycloaliphatic, or heteroalicyclic group.  Therefore, most of the compounds that have been prepared and tested bear a 2-chloroethyl group on N-1 and miscellaneous groups on N-3. The three disubstituted nitrosoureas shown below are undergoing extensive clinical trials.  They are N, N'-bis(2-chloroethyl)-N-nitrosourea (BCNU; NSC **409962**), N-(2-chloroethyl)-N'-cyclohexyl-N-nitrosourea (CCNU; NSC **79037**), and N-(2-chloroethyl)-N'-(<u>trans</u>-4-methylcyclohexyl)-N-nitrosourea (MeCCNU; NSC **95441**).

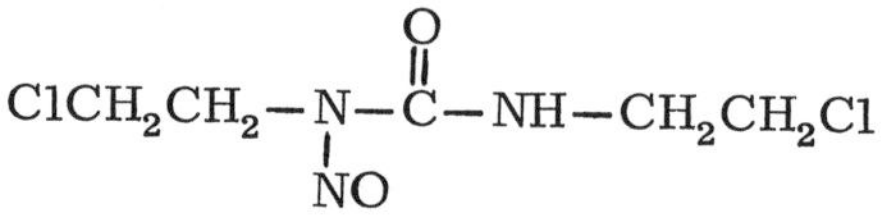

$$ClCH_2CH_2-\underset{\underset{NO}{|}}{N}-\overset{\overset{O}{\|}}{C}-NH-CH_2CH_2Cl$$

<u>BCNU ( NSC **409962**)</u>

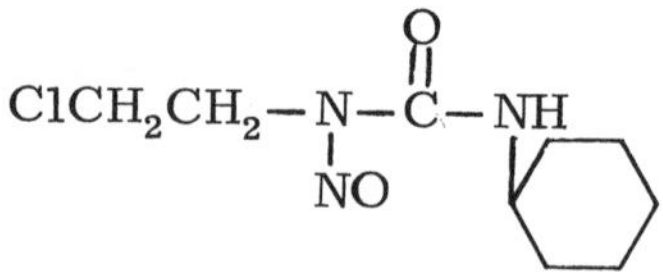

$$ClCH_2CH_2-\underset{\underset{NO}{|}}{N}-\overset{\overset{O}{\|}}{C}-NH$$

<u>CCNU (NSC **79037**)</u>

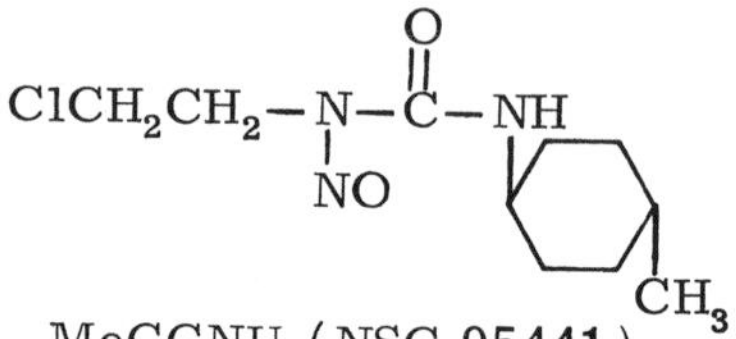

$$ClCH_2CH_2-\underset{\underset{NO}{|}}{N}-\overset{\overset{O}{\|}}{C}-NH$$

CH₃
<u>MeCCNU ( NSC **95441** )</u>

## Mode of Decomposition

It was hypothesized early that the observed biological effects of MNNG (**5**) and of MNU (**11**) were due to their decomposition at physiological conditions to yield diazomethane, which would then alkylate biological materials.  Subsequent studies have shown that alkylation of biological materials does in fact occur, but experiments with MNNG (**12**), MNU (**13**,**14**), and N-ethyl-N-nitrosourea (**15**) that were labeled with [14]C, [3]H, or [2]H in the methyl or ethyl group showed that methyl or ethyl groups of the alkylation products contained the same ratios of isotopes as the parent compounds, and therefore a diazoalkane could <u>not</u> be an intermediate. This and other evidence is consistent with the intermediate formation (as shown below) of methanediazohydroxide, which then decomposes to generate a methyl cation.

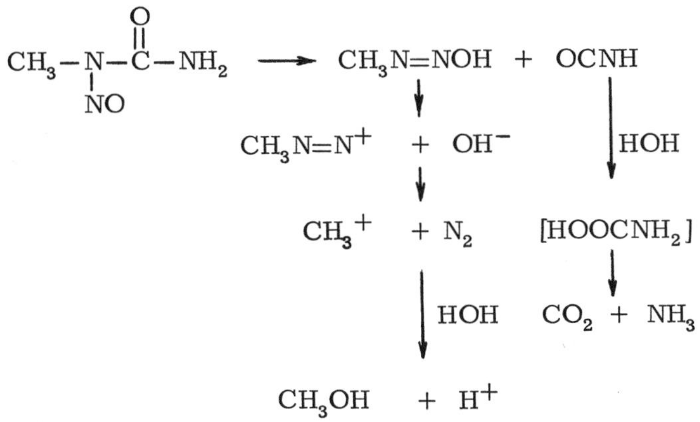

$$CH_3 - \underset{\underset{NO}{|}}{N} - \overset{\overset{O}{\|}}{C} - NH_2 \longrightarrow CH_3N{=}NOH \ + \ OCNH$$

$$CH_3N{=}N^+ \ + \ OH^- \qquad HOH$$

$$CH_3^+ \ + \ N_2 \qquad [HOOCNH_2]$$

$$HOH \qquad CO_2 \ + \ NH_3$$

$$CH_3OH \ + \ H^+$$

By analogy with the decomposition of MNU, it would be expected that the decomposition of N-(2-chloroethyl)-N'-substituted-N-nitrosoureas would yield 2-chloroethanediazohydroxide and the corresponding isocyanate. The 2-chloroethanediazohydroxide would give rise to a 2-chloroethyl cation, which could combine with a hydroxide ion or water to form 2-chloroethanol. In 1967 Montgomery and co-workers (16) reported that decomposition of BCNU and of CCNU in water yielded primarily acetaldehyde rather than 2-chloroethanol. This suggested the intermediate generation of a vinyl cation rather than a 2-chloroethyl cation, and they suggested the following mechanistic sequence. By this scheme the loss of a proton and a chloride ion gives rise to an unstable oxazolidine intermediate, which then breaks down into ethylenediazohydroxide and an isocyanate. In contrast to BCNU, BFNU (N,N'-bis(2-fluoroethyl)-N-nitrosourea) decomposed in the normal manner to yield 2-fluoroethanol.

$$ClCH_2CH_2-\underset{NO}{\underset{|}{N}}-\overset{O}{\overset{||}{C}}-NHR \longrightarrow ClCH_2CH_2-\underset{NO}{\underset{|}{N}}-\overset{O^{\ominus}}{\overset{|}{C}}=NR + H^{\oplus}$$

$$CH_2=CHN=NOH + OCNR$$

$$CH_2=CHN=N^{\oplus} + OH^{\ominus}$$

$$CH_3CHO \longleftarrow [CH_2=CHOH] + H^{\oplus} \overset{H_2O}{\longleftarrow} CH_2=CH^{\oplus} + N_2$$

In 1974 Colvin, Cowens, Brundrett, Kramer, and Ludlum (17) studied the decomposition of [14]C-labeled BCNU in phosphate buffer at pH 7.4 and found that contrary to the results of Montgomery et al. 63% of the identified volatile material was 2-chloroethanol and 31% was acetaldehyde; other volatile compounds included dichloroethane and vinyl chloride. They also obtained evidence (18) for the formation of a 2-chloroethyl cation from CCNU. Reed et al. (19) reported evidence supporting the formation of the 2-chloroethyl cation and of 2-chloroethanol when CCNU or MeCCNU decomposes in buffered aqueous solutions, and they proposed the following mechanism, which involves base catalysis. Montgomery and co-workers presented (20) the results of additional studies of the decomposition of six N-(2-chloroethyl)-N'-substituted-N-nitrosoureas (including BCNU and CCNU) in both water and buffered solutions, and they concluded that it is likely that at physiological conditions both of the above modes of decomposition occur. The relative extents of the two modes depend upon whether or not the solution is buffered at or near physiological pH. In unbuffered solutions the major volatile product was acetaldehyde, and only very small quantities of 2-chloroethanol were

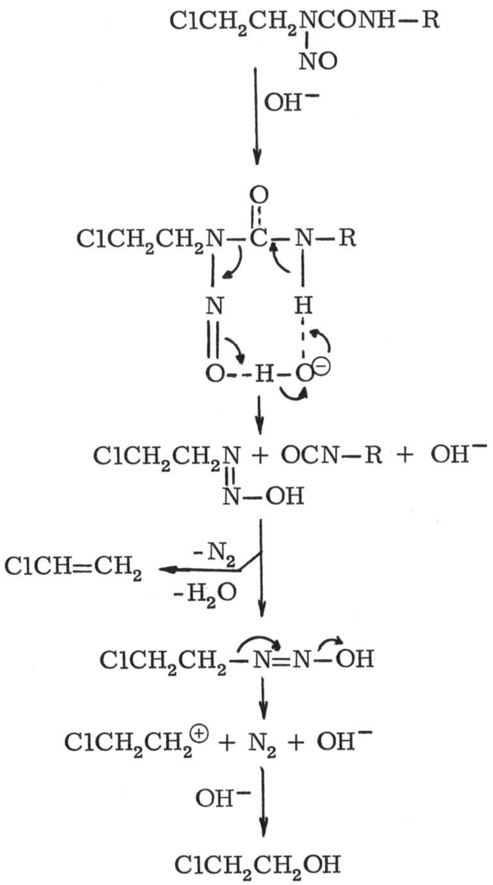

$$ClCH_2CH_2\underset{\underset{NO}{|}}{N}CONH-R$$

$$\downarrow OH^-$$

$$ClCH_2CH_2\underset{\underset{N}{|}}{N}-\overset{\overset{O}{||}}{C}-\underset{\underset{H}{|}}{N}-R$$

$$\overset{||}{O}--H-\overset{\ominus}{O}$$

$$ClCH_2CH_2\underset{\underset{N-OH}{||}}{N} + OCN-R + OH^-$$

$$ClCH=CH_2 \xleftarrow[-H_2O]{-N_2} \downarrow$$

$$ClCH_2CH_2-N=N-OH$$

$$\downarrow$$

$$ClCH_2CH_2^{\oplus} + N_2 + OH^-$$

$$OH^- \downarrow$$

$$ClCH_2CH_2OH$$

formed.  In buffered solutions much less acetaldehyde and much more 2-chloroethanol were produced.  The 2-chloroethyl cation can be a precursor of acetaldehyde ($\underline{20}$), so part of the acetaldehyde might be formed by this pathway in addition to its formation via the vinyl cation.

The isocyanates that are generated upon the decomposition of the nitrosoureas can react with water to form carbamic acids, which in turn decompose to yield carbon dioxide and the corresponding amines.  If the concentration and the pH of the mixture are suitable, the amine may react with the isocyanate to yield the symmetrical urea.

$$RNCO \xrightarrow{H_2O} [RNHCOOH] \longrightarrow RNH_2 + CO_2$$

$$RNH-\underset{\underset{O}{\|}}{C}-NHR$$

If nucleophiles (including biological materials) other than hydroxyl ion are present during the decomposition of the nitrosourea the carbonium ions might alkylate them. Also if compounds containing active hydrogen atoms are present they might react with the isocyanate by a carbamoylation reaction. Either alkylation or carbamoylation (or both) of biological materials might cause the observed physiological effects of these agents. In the special cases where the substituent upon N-3 is a 2-haloethyl group the amine formed via the carbamic acid would be a 2-haloethylamine, which in itself might serve as an alkylating agent; this would be the case for BCNU.

## Products of Alkylation

Utilizing CCNU labeled with [14]C in the 2-chloroethyl group, Cheng, Fujimura, Grunberger, and Weinstein (21) observed the binding of the isotope to poly U, poly A, poly $(G_1 U_3)$, poly G, poly C, tRNA, DNA, albumin, histone, ribonuclease A, and cytochrome C upon incubating mixtures in buffered solutions, pH 7.2 at 37°. They also observed that the [14]C was bound to the RNA, DNA, and protein of leukemia L1210 cells following incubation of the CCNU with cells in vitro, and Connors and Hare (22) similarly observed the binding of [14]C to RNA, DNA, and protein upon incubation of this labeled agent with murine TLX5 ascites cells. Following the administration of the CCNU to mice bearing the ascitic form of the leukemia L1210, [14]C was associated with the three types of macromolecules.

Kramer, Fenselau, and Ludlum (23) have identified an alkylated base that was formed upon exposure of a polynucleotide to a N-(2-chloroethyl)-N-nitrosourea. These investigators incubated [2-chloroethyl-[14]C]BCNU with poly C, and after acid hydrolysis of the polymer they isolated two products which they identified as 3-(2-hydroxyethyl) CMP (I) and 3,$N^4$-ethano-CMP (II). Both of these compounds upon decomposition yielded 3-(2-hydroxyethyl)-UMP (III). They suggest that a 3-(2-chloroethyl)cytosine moiety may have been an intermediate product in the formation of the isolated products.

I                              III                              II

      Because of the well-known mutagenic and carcinogenic activities of MNU and N-ethyl-N-nitrosourea (ENU) (see below) the alkylation of nucleic acids by these agents has been studied by a number of investigators. Table I lists the alkylated bases that have been isolated and identified following the treatment of deoxyguanosine (**24**), DNA (**25, 26, 27, 28, 29**), tRNA (**30**), TMV-RNA (**31**), and bacteriophage R17 (**32**). The products that have been isolated after incubating intact cells with MNU or ENU are given in Table II. In most instances, 7-MeGua was formed in much greater quantity than the other methylated bases. The evidence (**26, 33**) indicates that the extent of formation of phosphotriesters is greater than that of most of the alkylated bases but still much less, with two exceptions (**29, 31**), than that of 7-MeGua. Table III lists the alkylated bases that have been isolated from nucleic acids of various tissues following the administration of MNU or ENU to experimental animals.

Table I

Products Isolated after Incubation of Various Materials with MNU or ENU

| Deoxyguanosine (24) | DNA (25, 26, 27) | DNA (28) | DNA (29) | t-RNA (30) | TMV-RNA (31) | Bacteriophage B17 (32) |
|---|---|---|---|---|---|---|
| $O^6$-MedGuo | $O^6$-MedGuo | $O^6$-MeGua | $O^6$-EtGua | $O^6$-MeGua | $O^6$-EtGua | $O^6$-MeGua |
| $O^6$-EtdGuo | 7-MeGua | 7-MeGua | 7-EtGua | 7-MeGua | 7-EtGua | 7-MeGua |
|  | 3-MeGua |  | 3-EtGua |  | 3-EtGua | 3-MeGua |
|  | 1-MedAdo | 1-MeAde | 1-EtAde | 1-MeAde | 1-EtAde | 1-MeAde |
|  | 3-MeAde | 3-MeAde | 3-EtAde | 3-MeAde | 3-EtAde | 3-MeAde |
|  | 7-MeAde | 7-MeAde | 7-EtAde | 7-MeAde | 7-EtAde |  |
|  | 3-MedCyd |  | 3-EtCyt | 3-MeCyt | 3-EtCyt | 3-MeCyt |
|  | 3-MedThd | — | 3-EtThy | — |  |  |
|  | $O^4$-MedThd |  |  |  |  |  |
|  | Xp(Me)Y | — | Phosphotriester (Indirect evidence) | — | Phosphotriester (Indirect evidence) | Phosphotriester (Indirect evidence) |

Table II
Products Isolated after Incubating Cells with MNU or ENU

| HeLa Cells (29) | L-Cells (33) | E. Coli (15) |
|---|---|---|
| $O^6$-EtGua<br>7-EtGua<br>3-EtGua | $O^6$-MeGua<br>7-MeGua | $O^6$-EtGua<br>7-EtGua |
| 1-EtAde<br>3-EtAde<br>7-EtAde | 3-MeAde | 3-EtAde |
| 3-EtCyt | | |
| 3-EtThy | | |
| Phospho-triester (Indirect evidence) | Phospho-triester (Indirect evidence) | |

Table III
Products Isolated from Tissues of Experimental Animals
Following Administration of MNU or ENU
(13, 34-44)

| | |
|---|---|
| $O^6$-MeGua | $O^6$-EtGua |
| 7-MeGua | 7-EtGua |
| | 3-EtGua |
| 3-MeAde | 3-EtAde |
| | 7-EtAde |

Experiments have shown that the relative extents of alkylation of the various positions on the various bases of DNA and RNA differ for several biological alkylating agents. Comparison of the sites and extents of alkylation of DNA by methyl methanesulfonate, ethyl methanesulfonate, isopropyl methanesulfonate, and MNU (27) and by diethyl sulfate, ethyl methanesulfonate, and ENU (29) showed that MNU and ENU caused relatively more alkylation of the $O^6$-position of guanine than the other agents. Similar results were obtained in experiments with RNA and: diethyl sulfate, ethyl methanesulfonate, and ENU (31); dimethyl sulfate, methyl methanesulfonate, MNU, and MNNG (32); and dimethyl sulfate, MNU, and MNNG (45); MNU and MNNG yielded similar results. The nitrosoureas also caused the formation of larger quantities of phosphotri-esters than the other agents (29, 31, 32). There is also evidence that ethyl methanesulfonate alkylates the $O^6$-position of guanine

moieties more extensively than methyl methanesulfonate and
that ENU alkylates this position more than MNU (<u>24</u>, <u>27</u>, <u>46</u>).
Lawley (<u>27</u>, <u>46</u>) has pointed out that these results are consistent with the Swain-Scott factors for the alkylating agents and
the nucleophilicities of the sites on the bases.  The relationships of these differences to biological effects will be mentioned
below.
     Consideration of the multiplicity of alkylation products
listed above for MNU and ENU makes it evident that much work
remains to be done to isolate and identify alkylation products
obtained with N-(2-chloroethyl)-N-nitrosoureas.  The task may
be more difficult, if the alkylation products are 2-chloroethyl
amines or sulfides, because these compounds themselves might
be chemically active as alkylating agents.

## Products of Carbamoylation

     Soon after the initiation of studies with nitrosoureas it
was recognized that carbamoylation of biological materials
might play a role in causing the physiological effects of the
agents (<u>16</u>, <u>47</u>).  In 1968 we reported (<u>48</u>) that 2-chloroethyl
isocyanate was as effective as BCNU in decreasing the DNA
nucleotidyltransferase activity of crude preparations from
leukemia L1210 cells, and we obtained evidence (<u>49</u>) that carbamoylation of the $\epsilon$-amino group of lysine moieties occurred
when BCNU was incubated with histone.  Oliverio and co-workers reported (<u>50</u>, <u>51</u>) that following the administration of CCNU
to dogs and monkeys the cyclohexyl portion, but not the
2-chloroethyl portion, of the parent compound was bound to
the plasma protein.  Weinstein and collaborators (<u>21</u>, <u>52</u>)
observed that the cyclohexyl portion of CCNU was extensively
bound to globulin, ribonuclease A, cytochrome C, histone,
albumin, and polylysine (in increasing order) and to proteins
of L1210 cells, and hydrolysis of the latter four treated materials yielded $N^6$-cyclohexylcarbamoyllysine.  We have recently
observed (<u>53</u>) that at physiological conditions the carbamoylation of the $N^2$ of lysine occurs more extensively than carbamoylation of $N^6$.  Table IV shows the relative amounts of
products obtained when a mixture of equimolar quantities of
CCNU and lysine was incubated in 0.1 M phosphate buffer at 37°.

Table IV
Relative Quantities of Products Formed Upon Incubating a
Mixture of L-[U-$^{14}$C]Lysine and CCNU

| Product | Relative Quantity |
|---|---|
| $N^2$-(Cyclohexylcarbamoyl)lysine | 1.00 |
| $N^6$-(Cyclohexylcarbamoyl)lysine | 0.38 |
| $N^2$, $N^6$-Di(cyclohexylcarbamoyl)lysine | 0.09 |

Experiments with other $\alpha$-amino acids and with dipeptides also demonstrated the carbamoylation of $N^2$ of amino acids and of terminal amino groups of peptides.  Incubation of a mixture of insulin and CCNU, and hydrolysis of the reaction product yielded N-cyclohexylcarbamoylglycine and N-cyclohexylcarbamoylphenylalanine, which shows that carbamoylation of the amino terminal moieties occurred.  We did not detect any $N^6$-cyclohexylcarbamoyllysine, which would have been indicative of carbamoylation of the single lysine moiety present in the molecule, but it is emphasized that we did not diligently seek $N^6$-cyclohexylcarbamoyllysine.

We have observed (**53**) that even at room temperature cyclization of the 2-chloroethylcarbamoylamino groups can occur to form oxazolinyl groups as shown for $N^6$-(2-chloroethylcarbamoyl)lysine.  Similar cyclization occurs if the

$$\underset{\text{NH}_3{}^+}{\text{ClCH}_2\text{CH}_2\text{NH}\overset{\overset{\text{O}}{\|}}{\text{C}}\text{NHCH}_2\text{CH}_2\text{CH}_2\text{CHCOO}^-} \longrightarrow$$

$$\underset{\text{NH}_3{}^+}{\overset{\text{H}_2\text{C}-\text{O}}{\underset{\text{H}_2\text{C}-\text{N}}{}}\text{CNHCH}_2\text{CH}_2\text{CH}_2\text{CH}_2\text{CHCOO}^-}$$

2-chloroethylcarbamoyl group is on $N^2$ of an amino acid.  The oxazolinyl group is more basic than the 2-chloroethylcarbamoylamino group, and the oxazolinyl compound migrates electrophoretically similarly to the parent amino acid.  This cyclization is analogous to that which occurs when 1,3-bis(2-chloroethyl)urea (**54**) or chloroethylbiurets (**55**) are heated in boiling water.  Under physiological conditions that permit cyclization of 2-chloroethylcarbamoyl groups, there is no evidence of alteration of cyclohexylcarbamoyl groups.  Therefore, proteins carbamoylated upon treatment with BCNU might have different biochemical properties from those carbamoylated upon treatment with CCNU and other nitrosoureas.

There is evidence that carbamoylation of nucleic acids might occur to a small extent.  Utilizing [cyclohexyl-$^{14}$C]CCNU (**21**) and [carbonyl-$^{14}$C]CCNU (**52**) in experiments with isolated nucleic acids and with intact L1210 cells the Columbia University group detected a relatively minute quantity of $^{14}$C associated with RNA and with DNA in comparison to the quantity associated with proteins under the same conditions.  Serebryanyi and co-workers (**56**) incubated a mixture of [carbonyl-$^{14}$C]MNU with DNA and observed that the $^{14}$C became bound to the DNA.

Upon consideration of the relative nucleophilicities of phosphate, hydroxyl, and amino groups at pH 7, they suggested that carbamoylation would occur chiefly with the phosphate groups but carbamoylation of the bases might also occur. Upon conversion of the carbamoylated DNA to the corresponding apurinic acid a small amount of $^{14}C$ was retained. No carbamoylation product was identified. More recently Serebryanyi and Mnatsakanyan (57) have incubated adenosine or cytidine with MNU at physiological conditions and have obtained chromatographic and ultraviolet spectral data that are consistent with the formation of $N^6$-carbamoyladenosine and $N^4$-carbamoylcytidine.

## Metabolism of Nitrosoureas

There is evidence that certain nitrosoureas are altered by enzymatic metabolism to yield the products shown in Table V.

### Table V
### Products of Metabolism of Nitrosoureas

| Agent | System | Products | Reference |
|---|---|---|---|
| BCNU | Microsomal | N, N'-Bis(2-chloroethyl)-urea | (58) |
| BCNU | Liver cytosol | Unidentified | (58) |
| CCNU | Microsomal and in vivo | Ring-hydroxylated CCNU Cis-2 and/or trans-2 Trans-3 Cis-3 Trans-4 Cis-4 | (60, 61, 62) |

Hill et al. (58) observed that BCNU is converted to 1,3-bis(2-chloroethyl)urea by microsomal mixed-function oxidase that requires TPNH and oxygen. When the microsome preparation was replaced with a liver cytosol preparation, a product that has not been identified was obtained.

May, Boose, and Reed (59) and Hill, Kirk, and Struck (58) presented evidence that hydroxylation of the cyclohexyl ring occurs very rapidly when CCNU is incubated with a liver microsomal preparation in the presence of oxygen and TPNH. Reed and May (60, 61) identified five metabolites, which they obtained in vitro and in vivo and which are listed in the table. They did not specify the configuration of the 2-hydroxy derivative, but in a personal communication Dr. Reed stated that it is the cis-2-isomer. Hilton and Walker (62) have independently identified the two pairs of 3- and 4-isomers and the trans-2-isomer as products of in vitro incubation and also found them in the plasma of rats. Only the cis-4-isomer and the trans-4-isomer were found in human plasma following the intravenous

administration of CCNU; these isomers were present in approximately equal quantities (63).   The data of all of these groups
of investigators indicate that the rate of metabolic hydroxylation
exceeds the rate of chemical breakdown of CCNU, and therefore,
it is likely that the hydroxylated metabolites are intermediate
precursors of the therapeutically active moieties.   There is also
evidence (58, 59) that hydroxylation of MeCCNU occurs.   Because
of these facts the various hydroxylated compounds are being
synthesized (60, 64) and evaluated in chemotherapeutic trials.
The cis-4- and trans-4-isomers were more active against leukemia L1210 and more toxic than CCNU (64).

Cowens, Brundrett, and Colvin (65) observed that N-(2-
chloroethyl)-N', N-dimethyl-N-nitrosourea is stable in aqueous
solution and is inactive against L1210 leukemia in vitro but is
active against this leukemia in vivo.   This suggests that metabolic alteration gives rise to a more labile nitrosourea.

The types and extents of metabolic alteration of nitrosoureas bearing other types of substituents on N-3 are not known,
and the relevance of the known alterations to therapeutic effec-
tiveness is not presently known.   It can be expected, however,
that metabolism would alter the physical and chemical properties
of the parent compounds, and therefore one must exercise
caution in inferring the transposition of results obtained in
vitro to an in vivo situation.

Reed and May (60) also observed that a major urinary
metabolite of CCNU in mice is thiodiacetic acid, which is evidence of thiol alkylation.   They suggest that the alkylation might
involve a 2-chloroethyl cation or 2-chloroacetaldehyde, which
could be formed upon enzymatic oxidation of 2-chloroethanol.

### Relationships of Physicochemical and Chemical Properties to Therapeutic Usefulness

One of the advantages that the most effective nitrosoureas
have over several other types of anticancer agents is the fact
that their degree of lipoid solubility permits them (or perhaps
their metabolically altered derivatives) to cross such interfaces
as the "blood-brain barrier" and thus kill neoplastic cells present
in the brain (7).   Hansch, Smith, Engle, and Wood (66) used
the octanol-water partition coefficients to study the relationship
of lipophilicity to activity against intracerebrally inoculated
L1210 cells, and Montgomery, Mayo, and Hansch (67) carried
out a similar study with subcutaneous Lewis lung carcinoma.
They found that there is an optimum range for the partition
coefficient.   While lipophilicity is surely an important factor in
determining the biological activity of the nitrosoureas, it seems
likely that ultimately the biological effects will depend upon the
alkylating and carbamoylating activities of the agents or their
metabolic derivatives.   Therefore we attempted (68) to relate

Table VI

$$R-\underset{\underset{NO}{|}}{N}-\overset{\overset{O}{\|}}{C}-NH-R'$$

| R | R' | $T_{0.5}$ (min)[a] | $A_{540}$[b] | dpm[c] | Marrow toxicity |
|---|---|---|---|---|---|
| $ClCH_2CH_2-$ | (cyclohexyl) | 53 | 0.520 | 42.000 | High (69) |
| $ClCH_2CH_2-$ | (cyclohexyl-OH) | -- | ----- | 16,438 | ------ |
| $ClCH_2CH_2-$ | (cyclohexyl, OAc, OH) | -- | ----- | 30,218 | ------ |
| $ClCH_2CH_2-$ | (cyclohexyl OAc) | 44 | 1.133 | 21,076 | High (70) |
| $ClCH_2CH_2-$ | (cyclohexyl OAc) | 49 | 1.106 | 42,789 | High (70) |
| $ClCH_2CH_2-$ | (sugar, $CH_2OH$, OH, OH, HO) | 21 | 2.35 | 824 | Low (71) |
| $ClCH_2CH_2-$ | (sugar, $CH_2OAc$, OAc, OAc, AcO) | 16 | 2.74 | 41,197 | Low (69) |

[a]Half-life in ethanol / phosphate buffer, (1/50), pH 7.4, 37°. It was necessary to initially dissolve some of the compounds in acetone, and in such instances equal volumes of acetone were added to the blanks.

[b]$A_{540}$ is a measure of the concentration of alkylated 4-(p-nitrobenzyl)pyridine in an ethyl acetate extract of a mixture of the nitrosourea and 4-(p-nitrobenzyl)pyridine in acetate buffer, pH 6.0, that had been incubated at 37° for 2 hr.

[c]The dpm is a measure of the radioactivity present in unidentified reaction products obtained upon incubating the nitrosourea with lysine-14C in phosphate buffer, pH 7.4, at 37° for 6 hr.

each of these three parameters, namely, partition coefficient, alkylating activity, and carbamoylating activity, and the summation of them to the therapeutic activity against i. p. L1210. Upon the basis of mathematical correlation we concluded that all three parameters are important. We suggested that the lipophilicity was a major factor because it determined the extent of delivery of the agent to the desired site, that a dominant influence of the carbamoylating activity might be associated with the whole animal toxicity of the agent, and that the alkylating activity is important in determining the therapeutic index. We stress that these assignments are merely suggestions, because it is quite difficult to obtain and properly evaluate data for a multifactor system such as this.

The possible relevance of carbamoylating activity to whole animal toxicity is suggested by a consideration of the data in Table VI, which lists the chemical half-lives, the alkylating activities, and the carbamoylating activities, which we have determined for several nitrosoureas, and the relative marrow toxicities that others have reported. CCNU, which has a high in vitro carbamoylating activity, has a high marrow toxicity (69), and therefore, by inference, one would assume that at least certain of the hydroxylated metabolic derivatives of CCNU would also be myelosuppressive. The data show that the carbamoylating activities of the cis-4 and trans-4-hydroxy compounds have lower, but still moderately high, carbamoylating activity, as do also the acetylated cis-2 and trans-2-hydroxy compounds. Although the relevance of the in vitro data to the in vivo situation might be questionable, since it is quite possible that the acetyl groups are removed in vivo, these two compounds did have high marrow toxicity in vivo. Chlorozotocin [2-[3-(2-chloroethyl)-3-nitrosoureido]-2-deoxy-D-gluco-pyranose] (72), which has a high alkylating activity and a low carbamoylating activity, has a low marrow toxicity (71). The low marrow toxicity of the chlorozotocin tetraacetate along with the high in vitro carbamoylating activity is perhaps due to removal of the acetyl groups in vivo. In the N-methyl-N-nitrosourea series of compounds (73) the decrease in marrow toxicity parallels the decrease in carbamoylating activity (Table VII). Comparison such as this is being extended to analogs of chlorozotocin as they become available.

Schein et al. (74) observed that chlorozotocin was much less inhibitory than BCNU for DNA synthesis by human marrow in vitro which correlated with the differences in carbamoylating activity.

Table VII

$$R-N-\overset{\overset{\displaystyle O}{\|}}{\underset{\underset{\displaystyle NO}{|}}{C}}-NH-R'$$

| R | R' | $T_{0.5}$ (min)[a] | $A_{540}$[b] | dpm[c] | Marrow toxicity |
|---|---|---|---|---|---|
| $CH_3-$ | $-H$ | 7 | 0.356 | 10,892 | High (73) |
| $CH_3-$ | | 486 | 0.016 | 19,777 | ------ |
| $CH_3-$ | | 48 | 0.190 | 1,629 | Low (73) |

[a]Half-life in ethanol/phosphate buffer, (1/50), pH 7.4, 37°. It was necessary to initially dissolve some of the compounds in acetone, and in such instances equal volumes of acetone were added to the blanks.

[b]$A_{540}$ is a measure of the concentration of alkylated 4-(p-nitrobenzyl) pyridine in an ethyl acetate extract of a mixture of the nitrosourea and 4-(p-nitrobenzyl) pyridine in acetate buffer, pH 6.0, that had been incubated at 37° for 2 hr.

[c]The dpm is a measure of the radioactivity present in unidentified reaction products obtained upon incubating the nitrosourea with lysine-$^{14}$C in phosphate buffer, pH 7.4, at 37° for 6 hr.

Table VIII lists the half-lives, the alkylating activities, and the carbamoylating activities of a number of nitrosoureas that have been synthesized by Johnston and co-workers at Southern Research Institute (**8, 9, 10**). These properties were determined as described previously (**68**). Although the activities of a number of these compounds against L1210 leukemia (**8, 9, 10**), have been determined, the marrow toxicities of most of them have not yet been examined.

It is obvious that the substituents on both N and N' have great influences upon the properties of the compounds and that to a considerable degree one can obtain compounds with specified properties by the proper selection of substituents.

## Biochemical Effects

A number of studies (reviewed in **3**) have shown that BCNU, CCNU, MNU, and N-propyl-N-nitrosourea inhibit the synthesis of DNA, RNA, and protein *in vitro* and *in vivo*. At lower concentrations or lower doses the inhibition of the synthesis of DNA was usually greater than the inhibition of synthesis of RNA and of protein. At still lower doses, and even at early times after the administration of the higher doses, stimulation of macromolecular synthesis often occurred. Similar inhibitions of the synthesis of DNA, RNA, and protein have been reported for streptozotocin (**75**), and inhibition of synthesis of DNA by chlorozotocin (**71**) and by chlorozotocin tetraacetate (**69**) was observed.

Several studies to investigate the effects of nitrosoureas upon specific steps of macromolecular synthesis have been carried out. Incubation of crude cell-free preparations from L1210 cells with BCNU or CCNU caused decreases in the DNA nucleotidyltransferase activity of the preparations, but N-(2-chloroethyl)N-nitrosourea and MNU had much less effect (**48**). 2-Chloroethyl isocyanate caused as much decrease as BCNU or CCNU, and it was suggested that the apparent deactivation of the enzyme by BCNU and CCNU was due chiefly to the reactions of the isocyanates generated from them. In experiments with purified DNA polymerases I and II isolated from rat liver and hepatoma (**76**), BCNU, CCNU, MeCCNU, 2-chloroethyl isocyanate, and cyclohexyl isocyanate inhibited DNA polymerase II but did not affect the activity of DNA polymerase I. DNA polymerase II is also sensitive to thiol-blocking agents, but DNA polymerase I is not (**77**). Auxiliary data (**77**) led to the suggestion that enzyme I is a repair enzyme and enzyme II is a replicative enzyme. Preincubation of DNA with the nitrosoureas or isocyanates did not significantly decrease its template activity in the assay system (**48, 76**). Thus, it appears that the inhibition of replicative DNA synthesis might be due at least partially to carbamoylation of the replicative polymerase. In studies of the

TABLE VIII

PROPERTIES OF NITROSOUREAS

$$R-N-\overset{O}{\overset{\|}{C}}-NH-R'$$
$$\quad\ \ NO$$

| NSC No. | R | R' | Half-life [a] | | | Alkylating Activity [b] | | | Carbamoylating Activity [c] | |
|---|---|---|---|---|---|---|---|---|---|---|
| | | | $T_{0.5}$ (min) | n | SD | $A_{540}$ | n | SD | dpm | n |
| 23909 | $CH_3-$ | $-H$ | 7.0 | 9 | 0.8 | 0.356 | 4 | 0.081 | 10892 | 1 |
| 47547 | $ClCH_2CH_2-$ | $-H$ | 1.3 | 4 | 0.1 | >3.0 | 2 | – | 8858 | 1 |
| 409935 | $CH_3-$ | $-CH_2CH_2Cl$ | 254 | 12 | 21 | 0.020 | 2 | 0.010 | 8851 | 1 |
| 409962 | $ClCH_2CH_2-$ | $-CH_2CH_2Cl$ | 43 | – | – | 1.382 | 15 | 0.252 | 28716 | 1 |
| 91728 | $FCH_2CH_2-$ | $-CH_2CH_2F$ | – | – | – | 1.257 | 3 | 0.093 | 19777 | 3 |
| 79653 | $CH_3-$ | 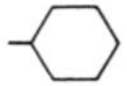 cyclohexyl | 486 | 12 | 46 | 0.016 | 2 | 0.004 | 19777 | 1 |
| 79037 | $ClCH_2CH_2-$ | 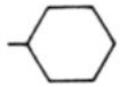 cyclohexyl | 52.5 | 3 | 0.8 | 0.520 | 28 | 0.091 | 42000 | (Arbitrary reference value) |
| 87974 | $FCH_2CH_2-$ | 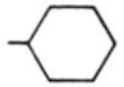 cyclohexyl | 68 | – | – | 0.640 | 7 | 0.070 | 49113 | 3 |
| 95441 | $ClCH_2CH_2-$ | 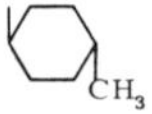 methylcyclohexyl ($CH_3$) | 53 | – | – | 0.520 | 12 | 0.071 | 38160 | 1 |
| 125649 | $FCH_2CH_2-$ | 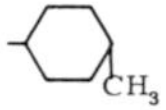 methylcyclohexyl ($CH_3$) | 58.6 | 4 | 4.4 | 0.610 | 4 | 0.017 | 49031 | 3 |
| 129967 | $ClCH_2CH_2-$ | 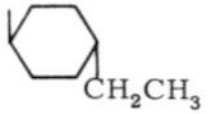 ethylcyclohexyl ($CH_2CH_3$) | 54 | – | – | 0.420 | 12 | 0.074 | 30206 | 1 |
| 129966 | $FCH_2CH_2-$ | 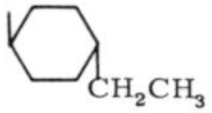 ethylcyclohexyl ($CH_2CH_3$) | 55.0 | 4 | 3.3 | 0.568 | 4 | 0.022 | 31789 | 2 |

| | | | $T_{0.5}$ | n | SD | $A_{540}$ | n | SD | dpm | n |
|---|---|---|---|---|---|---|---|---|---|---|
| 132086 | $FCH_2CH_2-$ | 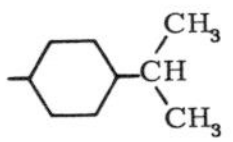 | — | — | — | 0.360 | 6 | 0.014 | 8910 | 2 |
| 132920 | $FCH_2CH_2-$ | 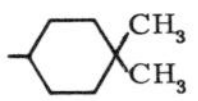 | 54.5 | 4 | 0.8 | 0.629 | 4 | 0.024 | 42449 | 2 |
| 93170 | $ClCH_2CH_2-$ | 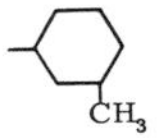 | — | — | — | 0.405 | 2 | 0.024 | — | — |
| 153174 | $ClCH_2CH_2-$ | 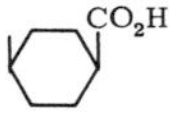 | 46.4 | 4 | 3.5 | 0.266 | 2 | — | — | — |
| 153175 | $ClCH_2CH_2-$ | 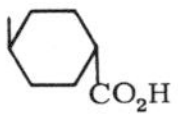 | 43.1 | 4 | 1.4 | 0.254 | 2 | — | — | — |
| 103548 | $ClCH_2CH_2-$ | 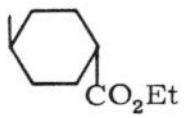 | 40.3 | 4 | 0.7 | 1.100 | 2 | 0.113 | — | — |
| 84954 | $ClCH_2CH_2-$ | 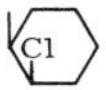 | 38 | — | — | 1.266 | 16 | 0.270 | 16367 | 2 |
| 88104 | $ClCH_2CH_2-$ | 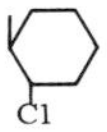 | 41 | — | — | 1.330 | 12 | 0.297 | 31157 | 2 |
| 95987 | $ClCH_2CH_2-$ | 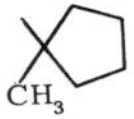 | — | — | — | 0.128 | 2 | 0.004 | — | — |
| 85998 | $CH_3-$ | 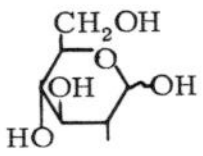 | 48.2 | 5 | 3.5 | 0.190 | 4 | 0.074 | 1629 | 4 |

TABLE VIII (*continued*)

| No. | R | Structure | $T_{0.5}$ | n | SD | $A_{540}$ | n | SD | dpm | n |
|---|---|---|---|---|---|---|---|---|---|---|
| 174793 | $CH_3CH_2-$ | [structure] | 45.9 | 3 | 2.3 | — | — | — | — | — |
| 178248 | $ClCH_2CH_2-$ | [structure] | 21.1 | 6 | 1.2 | 2.350 | 4 | 0.326 | 824 | 3 |
| 114460 | $ClCH_2CH_2-$ | [structure] | 16.1 | 4 | 0.8 | 2.740 | 4 | 0.048 | 41197 | 2 |
| 204818 | $ClCH_2CH_2-$ | [structure] | 48.5 | 4 | 0.9 | 1.106 | 4 | 0.062 | 42789 | 2 |
| 204817 | $ClCH_2CH_2-$ | [structure] | 43.7 | 4 | 1.3 | 1.133 | 4 | 0.072 | 21076 | 2 |
| 88106 | $ClCH_2CH_2-$ | [structure] | — | — | — | 0.647 | 2 | 0.016 | — | — |
| 93492 | $FCH_2CH_2-$ | [structure] | 55.7 | 4 | 3.0 | 0.853 | 2 | 0.068 | — | — |
| 129968 | $ClCH_2CH_2-$ | [structure] | 48 | — | — | 0.547 | 12 | 0.171 | 18625 | 1 |
| 132921 | $ClCH_2CH_2-$ | [structure] | 47.9 | 4 | 3.5 | 0.633 | 4 | 0.034 | 34968 | 2 |
| 110800 | $ClCH_2CH_2-$ | [structure] | 61.3 | 4 | 2.5 | 1.339 | 4 | 0.110 | 15730 | 2 |

| | n | dpm | SD | n | $A_{540}$ | SD | n | $T_{0.5}$ | Structure | Side chain | Number |
|---|---|---|---|---|---|---|---|---|---|---|---|
| | 2 | 17085 | 0.197 | 4 | 1.840 | 3.5 | 4 | 59.8 | | $FCH_2CH_2-$ | 121249 |
| | 1 | 10065 | 0.320 | 4 | 1.854 | 1.9 | 5 | 26.4 | | $ClCH_2CH_2-$ | 95466 |
| | 1 | 27345 | 0.093 | 2 | 1.142 | 1.3 | 5 | 49.1 | | $ClCH_2CH_2-$ | 103534 |
| | — | — | — | 2 | 1.351 | — | — | — | | $FCH_2CH_2-$ | 114459 |
| | 1 | 10866 | — | 12 | $>3.0$ | — | — | 19 | | $FCH_2CH_2-$ | 106767 |
| | 1 | 11476 | 0.117 | 5 | 2.369 | 0.3 | 4 | 22.4 | | $ClCH_2CH_2-$ | 105763 |
| | 1 | 13566 | 0.215 | 12 | 2.097 | — | — | 34 | | $FCH_2CH_2-$ | 132085 |
| | 1 | 13983 | 0.286 | 12 | 1.818 | — | — | 33 | | $ClCH_2CH_2-$ | 128303 |
| | 1 | 0 | — | 2 | $>3.0$ | 1.1 | 6 | 9.1 | | $FCH_2CH_2-$ | 136900 |
| | 1 | 175 | — | 2 | $>3.0$ | 1.9 | 4 | 8.3 | | $FCH_2CH_2-$ | 136902 |
| | 1 | 36652 | — | 2 | 0.006 | 0.2 | 4 | 5.6 | | | 80590 |

TABLE VIII (continued)

| Compound | Structure | $T_{0.5}$ | n | SD | $A_{540}$ | n | SD | dpm | n |
|---|---|---|---|---|---|---|---|---|---|
| 87426 | (chlorocyclohexyl) Cl | 8.1 | 4 | 1.8 | 0 | 1 | — | 9776 | 1 |
| 95462 | $ClCH_2CH-CH_3CH_2$ / $-CHCH_2Cl\ CH_2CH_3$ | 14.7 | 4 | 0.6 | 0.301 | 1 | — | 25143 | 1 |
| 82190 | $CH_3CH_2-$ / $-CH_2CH_3$ | 202 | 3 | 5 | 0 | 1 | — | 13733 | 1 |
| 95465 | $ClCHCH_2- CH_3$ / $-CH_2CHCl\ CH_3$ | 41.3 | 4 | 1.7 | 0.040 | 1 | — | 10287 | 1 |
| 74705 | $HO_2C(CH_2)_3-$ / $-(CH_2)_3CO_2H$ | 286 | 3 | 7 | 0 | 1 | — | 28391 | 1 |
| 95460 | $ClCHCH_2- CH_3$ (cyclohexyl) | 52.8 | 4 | 2.1 | 0.013 | 1 | — | 26272 | 1 |
| 67523 | (phenyl)$-CH_2$ / $-H$ | 3.0 | 4 | 0.3 | 0.161 | 1 | — | 6474 | — |
| 71911 | (phenyl)$-(CH_2)_2$ / $-H$ | 6.6 | 4 | 0.2 | 0.064 | 1 | — | 2308 | 1 |
| 72721 | $NC(CH_2)_2-$ / $-(CH_2)_2CN$ | 31.9 | 4 | 2.2 | 0.040 | 1 | — | 7006 | 1 |
| 93372 | $ClCH_2CH_2-$ / (cyclohexyl)$NH-C(=O)-N(NO)-CH_2CH_2Cl$ | — | — | — | 0.120 | 2 | 0.024 | — | — |
| 95459 | $FCH_2CH_2-$ / (cyclohexyl)$NH-C(=O)-N(NO)-CH_2CH_2F$ | — | — | — | 0.846 | 1 | — | — | — |

[a] Half-life in ethanol/phosphate buffer, (1/50), pH 7.4, 37°. It was necessary to initially dissolve some of the compounds in acetone, and in such instances equal volumes of acetone were added to the blanks.

[b] $A_{540}$ is a measure of the concentration of alkylated 4-(p-nitrobenzyl)pyridine in an ethyl acetate extract of a mixture of the nitrosourea and 4-(p-nitrobenzyl)pyridine in acetate buffer, pH 6.0, that had been incubated at 37° for 2 hr.

[c] The dpm is a measure of the radioactivity present in unidentified reaction products obtained upon incubating the nitrosourea with lysine-$^{14}$C in phosphate buffer, pH 7.4, at 37° for 6 hr.

repair of DNA that had been irradiated with X-rays (**78**) or
ultraviolet light (**79**) it was observed that BCNU and 2-chloro-
ethyl isocyanate interfered with the rejoining of broken strands
but not with the repair synthesis, which implies inhibition of
the ligase as a result of carbamoylation of it. These facts
suggest that the carbonium ions derived from the nitrosoureas
might alkylate DNA and the isocyanates derived from them
might interfere with the repair of the damaged DNA. One
might speculate that if nitrosoureas were used in combination
with other alkylating agents, both agents might cause alkylation
of DNA in an additive manner, and the generated isocyanate
might inhibit repair.

Incubation of DNA-dependent RNA polymerase from
Ehrlich ascites cells with MNU or N-propyl-N-nitrosourea
resulted in inhibition of the enzyme (**80**). Injection of these
agents into mice bearing Ehrlich ascites cells caused an
activation of the $Mg^{+2}$-dependent RNA synthesis by the isolated
nuclei from the ascites cells and at higher concentrations an
inhibition of the $Mn^{+2}/(NH_4)_2SO_4$-dependent RNA synthesis by
these nuclei (**81**). In studies with cultured leukemia L1210
cells it was found that BCNU inhibited the "processing" of
45S nucleolar RNA more readily than the synthesis of RNA,
and it also inhibited the "processing" or exit of high-molecular
weight RNA from the nucleoplasmic fraction (**82**). The
"processing" of nucleolar RNA was also inhibited by CCNU,
N-(2-fluoroethyl)-N'-cyclohexyl-N-nitrosourea, 2-chloroethyl
isocyanate, and cyclohexyl isocyanate, but not by MNU, N-(2-
chloroethyl)-N-nitrosourea, or streptozotocin. It was concluded that a carbamoylation reaction was responsible for
interference with the "processing". A comparison (**83**) of the
effects of nitrogen mustard (HN2), BCNU, and CCNU upon the
synthesis and "processing" of RNA by cultured HeLa cells
yielded the following results:

|  | HN2 | BCNU | CCNU |
|---|---|---|---|
| Inhibits formation of 45-S nRNA | Yes | No* | Yes |
| Inhibits "processing" of 45-S nRNA | No | Yes | Yes |
| Produces shortened HnRNA | Yes | No | No |
| Inhibits appearance of poly(A)-containing cytoplasmic RNA | Yes | Yes | No |

*Inhibition occurs after extended exposure.

Since each of these agents is an active anticancer agent, it is
obvious that bifunctionality, carbamoylation, and interference
with the formation and "processing" of RNA are not requisites
for anticancer activity.

A study (**84**) of the manner in which MNU interferes
with protein synthesis led to the conclusion that this agent can
damage polyribosomes and protein-soluble factors of the cell

sap, which leads to inhibition of polypeptide initiation and elongation. Other data (85) were interpreted to indicate that changes in the polyribosome profile induced by MNU reflects the mechanism of inhibition of protein synthesis rather than being a direct consequence of methylation of polysomal mRNA. MNU, ENU, and N-butyl-N-nitrosourea caused a significant stimulation of aminoacyl-tRNA complex formation but had no effect on the binding of nRNA to ribosomes (86).

The pharmacology of the nitrosoureas has been reviewed recently (4) and will not be discussed here, except to say that the half-lives of the compounds in the blood are very short, that the agents are widely distributed throughout the body without evidence of concentration in neoplastic tissues, and that the agents cross the "blood-brain barrier" and thus reach the brain and brain tumors.

As is the case with most anticancer agents, the reason(s) for the preferential cytotoxicity of the nitrosoureas for neoplastic tissues is not known. When rates of synthesis of DNA (87, 88, 89, 90) and of protein (84) are used as indicators of the "state of health" of various host and neoplastic tissues, it appears that both host and neoplastic tissues are damaged, but the host tissues recover the ability to synthesize these macromolecules more readily than the neoplastic tissues. The mechanisms of this recovery are not known, but they may include the repair of macromolecules and/or the repopulation of the tissues with viable cells with the accompanying loss of dead cells. It has been observed that deletion of methylated purines occurs following the treatment of Escherichi coli with ENU (15), of L-cells with MNU (33), and of mice with MNU (40, 42). Following the administration of [$C^{14}H_3$]MNU to mice bearing hepatomas, deletion of radioactivity from the DNA, RNA, protein, and lipids occurred more rapidly for spleen and liver than for the hepatoma (91). The relevance of these deletions to survival of the cells and tissues is considered below.

At minimal concentrations of streptozotocin and streptozotocin tetraacetate that were cytotoxic to cultured leukemia L1210 cells these agents did not significantly lower the levels of activity of thymidine kinase, thymidylate synthetase, and DNA polymerase (92). On the other hand, streptozotocin, MNU, and BCNU caused decreases in the observed activity of NAD glycohydrolase and the level of NAD in a variety of biological systems (reviewed in 3).

Biological Effects

Many published articles report that a number of nitrosoureas are active as carcinogenic, mutagenic, and teratogenic agents in a number of biological systems, and it is not deemed necessary to refer to each of those articles here. For the purpose of this review it is sufficient to state the nitrosoureas are quite potent in causing each of these biological effects. On the basis of the presently held dogmas of the role of nucleic acids in determining heritable traits in biological systems one might speculate that these effects derive from alteration of the nucleic acids of the cells that were exposed to the agents. The contents of Tables I, II, and III show that many alterations of the nucleic acids occur upon exposure to MNU and ENU, and one might ask whether the extent(s) of occurrence of one or more of these alterations correlates with the causation of one or more of the effects. A number of these investigators(13, 35, 36, 37, 38, 39) isolated and quantitatively determined only the 7-alkylguanines, and several of them (13, 36, 38, 39) concluded that there was no correlation between the extent of formation of 7-alkylguanine and carcinogenicity. Frei (34) detected and determined O⁶-MeGua and 3-MeAde in addition to 7-MeGua and suggested that this procedure might be useful in attempts to relate the formation of alkylated bases to carcinogenicity. This possibility is of interest, because it has been suggested by Loveless (24) that mutagenesis by these agents might be related to the formation of O⁶-alkylguanine moieties. Walker and Ewart (33) observed that following treatment of L-cells with MNU the deletion of 3-MeAde and 7-MeGua was more rapid than that of O⁶-MeGua. Goth and Rajewsky (44) found that after the treatment of rats with ENU, the deletion of 3-EtAde and 7-EtGua from liver and from brains occurred relatively rapidly, as did also the deletion of O⁶-EtGua from liver, but the deletion of O⁶-EtGua from brain occurred slowly. Kleihues and Margison (42) obtained analogous results with MNU for liver and brain and found that the rate of deletion of O⁶-MeGua from the DNA of kidney was intermediate between the rates for liver and brain. Frei and Lawley (40) compared the rates of deletion of alkylated purines from the DNA of bone marrow, small bowel, kidneys, liver, lungs, spleen, and thymus, but not the brain, of mice following the administration of MNU and found that 3-MeAde and 7-MeAde were deleted more rapidly than 3-MeGua, 7-MeGua, and O⁶-MeGua; there was little difference in the rates of deletion of 7-MeGua and O⁶-MeGua during the brief period (18 hours) of observation. Margison and Kleihues (43) observed that, when MNU was administered to rats in repeated small weekly doses that rather specifically gave rise to tumors of the nervous system, O⁶-MeGua accumulated in the DNA of the brain to a much greater extent than in the kidney, spleen, small intestine, and liver. Since the nervous system is the primary site of tumor formation following the administration of MNU and ENU (11, 93) and the kidney (93) is another frequent site, these results imply that the retention of O⁶-alkylguanine in the DNA might be conducive to carcinogenesis.

        The cause of the cytotoxicity of the nitrosoureas is not
known, and it seems likely that it might result from a combination of several mechanisms.  Verly (**94**) and Lawley et al.
(**95**) have suggested that the delayed inactivation of bacteriophage by monofunctional alkylating agents is related to the
presence of apurinic sites in the DNA following the elimination
of alkylated purines, and Lawley and Brooks (**96**) and Verly
and co-workers (**97**) have observed that the rate of elimination
of 3-alkyladenine is much greater than that of 7-alkylguanine.
The formation of and the subsequent hydrolysis of phospho-
triesters might also contribute to single-strand breaks of DNA
(**94**) and chain breaks of phage RNA (**32,98**) with resultant
phage deactivation.   These same mechanisms may contribute
to cytotoxicity in cells and tissues, but alkylation or carbamoylation of other critical cellular constituents might also be
contributing factors.
        Experiments have been performed to relate cytotoxicity
to sensitivity of mammalian cells in the various phases of the
cell cycle and to determine the effects of treatment with these
agents upon progression through the cell cycle.  The literature
prior to 1972 was reviewed (**3**), and it will not be repeated
here.   Several studies performed subsequent to that review
have confirmed and extended the previous conclusions.  Tobey
et al. (**99,100**) compared the effects of BCNU, CCNU, MeCCNU,
chlorozotocin, and streptozotocin in a single experimental
system and found the first four of these compounds had the
following similar effects:  (a) had little effect upon the progression of cells through $G_1$;  (b) caused a prolongation of S;
(c) caused cells to accumulate in late S or early $G_2$;  (d)
caused mitotic non-disjunction and polyploidy (cell enlargement);
(e) were more cytotoxic to non-cycling cells than to cycling
cells; and (f) caused an altered clonal morphology and growth
pattern in surviving cells.  Streptozotocin differed from the
other four compounds by causing less prolongation of S and less
accumulation of cells in late S and $G_2$ and by being more cytotoxic to cycling cells than to non-cycling cells at low concentrations.   Based upon another study Tobey (**101**) concluded that
chlorozotocin arrested cells in early $G_2$, streptozotocin arrested
them about one-third of the way through $G_2$, and BCNU and
CCNU arrested them about two-thirds of the way through $G_2$.
Other investigators (**102,103**) also observed that BCNU, CCNU,
and MeCCNU were more cytotoxic to plateau-phase or non-
dividing cells than to exponentially growing cells.  Hahn et al.
(**104**) suggested that the differential sensitivity of non-cycling
and cycling cells might partially be due to the anomolous binding
of BCNU to serum protein, but this is probably not the total
cause, because in the experiments of Tobey et al. serum was
present in the medium for both the cycling and the non-cycling
cells.   Contrary to the above observation for streptozotocin,

MNU prolonged the S phase without killing the cells (**105**).
These observations of the greater cytotoxic sensitivity of
plateau-phase cells and non-cycling cells to the nitrosoureas
differ from the observations with hematopoietic cells in vivo
(**106,107**) in which the rapidly proliferating cells were more
sensitive than the normal bone marrow.  However, non-pro-
liferating cells were sensitive to BCNU (**108**).  Although
cultured cells are sensitive to the cytotoxic effects of the nitrosoureas in all phases of the cell cycle (**75,109-113**), cells are
reported to be most sensitive in certain phases.  The most
sensitive phases have been reported variously for different
cell lines and different agents to be the $G_1$ / S boundary (**111**),
mid-S (**75,112**), and $G_2$ (**113**).

It was reported in 1963 (**114**) that streptozotocin is
diabetogenic, and many studies related to this property of the
compound and the disease it initiates have been performed (**115**).
There appears to be a considerable degree of structural specificity for elliciting diabetes, because although the ethyl analog
of streptozocin is diabetogenic, the 2-chloroethyl analog
(chlorozotocin) and chlorozotocin tetraacetate are not (**116**).
Also, MNU (**117**) and several analogs of streptozotocin in
which the glucosyl portion of the molecule is altered (**118**) are
also non-diabetogenic.  Streptozotocin causes a decrease in
the NAD content of pancreatic islets (**119,120,121**) perhaps by
reducing the tissue uptake of precursors and decreasing the
synthesis of NAD (**119**) and by inducing NAD degradation,
which can be prevented by inhibitors of NAD-glycohydrolases
(**120**).  The diabetogenic action is probably related to this
decrease in NAD concentration, since this action can be prevented by the administration of NAD (**122**).  MNU also
decreases the NAD content of pancreatic islets but to a lesser
extent than streptozotocin (**121**), and other nitrosoureas can
reduce the NAD content of various tissues (reviewed in **3**).
Therefore the glucose residue (**121**) in conjunction with the
presence of the methyl or ethyl group on the nitrosated nitrogen
(**116**) must cause additional specific cytotoxicity for the $\beta$-cells
of the pancreas.

Another observed effect of the nitrosoureas that might
be of potential practical usefulness is the prevention of the in
vitro sickling of red cells containing hemoglobin S (**123**) by
MNU, BCNU, and CCNU.  It appears likely that this prevention
results from the carbamoylation of the hemoglobin S, since
prevention also results when the cells are treated with 2-chloro-
ethyl isocyanate or cyclohexyl isocyanate and the treatment of
the cells or of mice with BCNU alters the electrophoretic
properties of the hemoglobin.  This reaction is probably analogous to the reaction of cyanate, which has undergone extensive
testing for this purpose, but the use of nitrosoureas as progenitors of isocyanates has the potential for accomplishing some
specificity of carbamoylation.

114

CANCER CHEMOTHERAPY

## Conclusions

It is always difficult to specifically define a chemical and / or biochemical mechanism by which a drug elicits a therapeutic response, and the difficulty is greater if the agent has a multiplicity of chemical activities and biochemical and physiological effects. Nevertheless, knowledge of the possible factors that may be involved in bringing about such a response can aid in rationally planning therapeutic regimens for use of the agents. It is hoped that the facts that have been presented in this review will be useful for such planning.

It is believed that the nitrosoureas have an established place in the cancer chemotherapy armamentarium. An expanding knowledge of the various aspects of their mechanisms of action should make possible a more effective use of the compounds already being used and serve as a guide in the preparation of other nitrosoureas that will have improved therapeutic indexes and more desirable physical and chemical properties.

## Literature Cited

1. Carter, S. K. , Schabel, F. M. , Jr. , Broder, L. E. , and Johnston, T. P. Adv. Cancer Res. (1972) 16, 273-332.
2. Wheeler, G. P. Biochem. Pharmacol. (1974) 23, Supplement No. 2, 225-232.
3. Wheeler, G. P. Handb. Exp. Pharmacol. (1975) 38/2, 65-84.
4. Oliverio, V. T. , Kohn, K. W. , and Wooley, P. V. Proc. of 11th Inter. Cancer Cong. , Florence, 1974 (1975) 5, 238-247.
5. Skinner, W. A. , Gram, H. F. , Greene, M. O. , Greenberg, J. , and Baker, B. R. J. Med. Pharm. Chem. (1960) 2, 299-333.
6. Hyde, K. A. , Acton, E. , Skinner, W. A. , Goodman, L. , Greenberg, J. , and Baker, B. R. J. Med. Pharm. Chem. (1962) 5, 1-14.
7. Skipper, H. E. , Schabel, F. M. , Jr. , Trader, M. W. , and Thomson, J. R. Cancer Res. (1961) 21, 1154-1164.
8. Johnston, T. P. , McCaleb, G. S. , and Montgomery, J. A. J. Med. Chem. (1963) 6, 669-681.
9. Johnston, T. P. , McCaleb, G. S. , Opliger, P. S. , and Montgomery, J. A. J. Med. Chem. (1966) 9, 892-911.
10. Johnston, T. P. , McCaleb, G. S. , Opliger, P. S. , Laster, W. R. , and Montgomery, J. A. J. Med. Chem. (1971) 14, 600-614.
11. Druckrey, H. , Ivanković, S. , and Preussmann, R. Z. Krebsforsch. (1965) 66, 389-408.

12. Süssmuth, R. , Haerlin, R. , and Lingens, F. Biochim. Biophys. Acta (1972) **269**, 276-286.
13. Lijinsky, W. , Garcia, H. , Keefer, L. , Loo, J. , and Ross, A. E. Cancer Res. (1972) **32**, 893-897.
14. Lawley, P. D. , and Shah, S. A. Chem. -Biol. Interact. (1973) **7**, 115-120.
15. Lawley, P. D. , and Warren, W. Chem. -Biol. Interact. (1975) **11**, 55-57.
16. Montgomery, J. A. , James, R. , McCaleb, G. S. , and Johnston, T. P. J. Med. Chem. (1967) **10**, 668-674.
17. Colvin, M. , Cowens, J. W. , Brundrett, R. B. , Kramer, B. S. , and Ludlum, D. B. Biochem. Biophys. Res. Commun. (1974) **60**, 515-520.
18. Colvin, M. , Cowens, J. W. , Brundrett, R. B. , and Ludlum, D. B. Fed. Proc. Fed. Am. Soc. Exp. Biol. (1975) **34**, 806.
19. Reed, D. J. , May, H. E. , Boose, R. B. , Gregory, K. M., and Beilstein, M. A. Cancer Res. (1975) **35**, 568-576.
20. Montgomery, J. A. , James, R. , McCaleb, G. S. , Kirk, M. C. , and Johnston, T. P. J. Med. Chem. (1975) **18**, 568-571.
21. Cheng, C. J. , Fujimura, S. , Grunberger, D. , and Weinstein, I. B. Cancer Res. (1972) **32**, 22-27.
22. Connors, T. A. , and Hare, J. R. Br. J. Cancer (1974) **30**, 477-480.
23. Kramer, B. S. , Fenselau, C. C. , and Ludlum, D. B. Biochem. Biophys. Res. Commun. (1974) **56**, 783-788.
24. Loveless, A. Nature (1969) **223**, 206-207.
25. Lawley, P. D. , Orr, D. J. , Shah, S. A. , Farmer, P. B., and Jarman, M. Biochem. J. (1973) **135**, 193-201.
26. Lawley, P. D. Chem. -Biol. Interact. (1973) **7**, 127-130.
27. Lawley, P. D. , Orr, D. J. , and Jarman, M. Biochem. J. (1975) **145**, 73-84.
28. Kirtikar, D. M. , and Goldthwait, D. A. Proc. Natl. Acad. Sci. USA (1974) **71**, 2022-2026.
29. Sun, L. , and Singer, B. Biochem. (1975) **14**, 1795-1802.
30. Pegg, A. E. Chem. -Biol. Interact. (1973) **6**, 393-406.
31. Singer, B. , and Fraenkel-Conrat, H. Biochemistry (1975) **14**, 772-782.
32. Shooter, K. V. , House, R. , Shah, S. A. , and Lawley, P. D. Biochem. J. (1974) **137**, 303-312.
33. Walker, I. G. , and Ewart, D. F. Mutat. Res. (1973) **19**, 331-341.
34. Frei, J. U. Int. J. Cancer (1971) **7**, 436-442.
35. Swann, P. F. , and Magee, P. N. Biochem. J. (1968) **110**, 39-47.
36. Krüger, F. W. , Ballweg, H. , and Maier-Borst, W. , Experientia (1968) **24**, 592-593.
37. Serebryanyi, A. M. , Smotryaeva, M. A. , and Kruglyakova, K. E. Izv. Akad. Nauk SSSR, Ser. Biol. (1969) **4**, 607-608.

38. Wunderlich, V. , and Tetzlaff, I.  Arch. Geschwulstforsch.
    (1970) 35, 251-258.
39. Goth, R. , and Rajewsky, M. F.  Cancer Res. (1972) 32,
    1501-1505.
40. Frei, J. V. , and Lawley, P. D.  Chem. -Biol. Interact.
    (1975) 10, 413-427.
41. Kleihues, P. , Stavrou, D. , Scharrer, E. , and Bücheler,
    J. Z. Krebsforsch. Klin. Onkol. (1973) 80, 317-322.
42. Kleihues, P. , and Margison, G. P. J. Natl. Cancer Inst.
    (1974) 53, 1839-1841.
43. Margison, G. P. , and Kleihues, P.  Biochem. J. (1975)
    148, 521-525.
44. Goth, R. , and Rajewsky, M. F. Proc. Natl. Acad. Sci.
    USA (1974) 71, 639-643.
45. Lawley, P. D. , and Shah, S. A.  Biochem. J. (1972)
    128, 117-132.
46. Lawley, P. D. Mutat. Res. (1974) 23, 283-295.
47. Wheeler, G. P. Cancer Res. (1962) 22, 651-688.
48. Wheeler, G. P. , and Bowdon, B. J.  Cancer Res. (1968)
    28, 52-59.
49. Bowdon, B. J. , and Wheeler, G. P. Proc. Am. Assoc.
    Cancer Res. (1971) 12, 67.
50. Oliverio, V. T. , Vietzke, W. M. , Williams, M. K. , and
    Adamson, R. H. Proc. Am. Assoc. Cancer Res. (1968)
    9, 56.
51. Oliverio, V. T. , Vietzke, W. M. , Williams, M. K. , and
    Adamson, R. H. Cancer Res. (1970) 30, 1330-1337.
52. Schmall, B. , Cheng, C. J. , Fujimura, S. , Gersten, N. ,
    Grunberger, D. , and Weinstein, I. B. Cancer Res. (1973)
    33, 1921-1924.
53. Wheeler, G. P. , Bowdon, B. J. , and Struck, R. F.
    Cancer Res. (In press).
54. Kreling, M. -E. , and McKay, A. F. Can. J. Chem. (1959)
    37, 504-505.
55. Johnston, T. P. , and Opliger, P. S. J. Med. Chem. (1967)
    10, 675-681.
56. Serebryanyi, A. M. , Smotryaeva, M. A. , Kruglyakova,
    K. E. , and Kostyanovskii, R. G. Dokl. Akad. , Nauk SSSR
    (1969) 185, 847-849.
57. Serebryanyi, A. M. , and Mnatsakanyan, R. M. FEBS
    Lett. (1972) 28, 191-194.
58. Hill, D. L. , Kirk, M. C. , and Struck, R. F. Cancer Res.
    (1975) 35, 296-301.
59. May, H. E. , Boose, R. , and Reed, D. J. Biochem. Bio-
    phys. Res. Commun. (1974) 57, 426-433.
60. Reed, D. J. , and May, H. E. Life Sciences (1975) 16,
    1263-1270.
61. Reed, D. J. Proc. Am. Assoc. Cancer Res. (1975) 16, 92.

62. Hilton, J. , and Walker, M. D.  Biochem. Pharmacol. (In press).
63. Hilton, J. , and Walker, M. D.  Proc. Am. Assoc. Cancer Res. (1975) 16, 103.
64. Johnston, T. P. , McCaleb, G. S. , and Montgomery, J. A. J. Med. Chem. (1975) 18, 634-637.
65. Cowens, W. , Brundrett, R. , and Colvin, M.  Proc. Am. Assoc. Cancer Res. (1975) 16, 100.
66. Hansch, C. , Smith, N. , Engle, R. , and Wood, H. Cancer Chemother. Rept. Part 1 (1972) 56, 443-456.
67. Montgomery, J. A. , Mayo, J. G. , and Hansch, C. J. Med. Chem. (1974) 17, 477-480.
68. Wheeler, G. P. , Bowdon, B. J. , Grimsley, J. A. , and Lloyd, H. H.  Cancer Res. (1974) 34, 194-200.
69. Schein, P. S. , McMenamin, M. G. , and Anderson, T. Cancer Res. (1973) 33, 2005-2009.
70. Schmidt, L. H.  Unpublished data.
71. Anderson, T. , McMenamin, M. G. , and Schein, P. S. Cancer Res. (1975) 35, 761-765.
72. Johnston, T. P. , McCaleb, G. S. , and Montgomery, J. A. J. Med. Chem. (1975) 18, 104-106.
73. Schein, P. S.  Cancer Res. (1969) 29, 1226-1232.
74. Schein, P. , Bull, J. , McMenamin, M. , and Macdonald, J. Proc. Am. Assoc. Cancer Res. (1975) 16, 122.
75. Bhuyan, B. K. , Fraser, T. J. , Buskirk, H. H. , and Neil, G. L.  Cancer Chemother. Rept. Part 1, (1972) 56, 709-720.
76. Baril, B. B. , Baril, E. F. , Laszlo, J. , and Wheeler, G. P.  Cancer Res. (1975) 35, 1-5.
77. Baril, E. F. , Jenkins, M. D. , Brown, O. E. , Laszlo, J. , and Morris, H. P.  Cancer Res. (1973) 33, 1187-1193.
78. Kann, H. E. , Jr. , Kohn, K. W. , and Lyles, J. M.  Cancer Res. (1974) 34, 398-402.
79. Fornace, A. J. , Jr. , Kohn, K. W. , and Kann, H. E. , Jr. Proc. Am. Assoc. Cancer Res. (1975) 16, 128.
80. Gorbacheva, L. B. , Mitskevich, L. G. , and Kukushkina, G. V.  Stud. Biophys. (1972) 31/32, 437-446.
81. Mitskevich, L. G. , Roset, E. G. , Kukushkina, G. V. , and Gorbacheva, L. B.  Biokhimiya (1972) 37, 851-854.
82. Kann, H. E. , Jr. , Kohn, K. W. , Widerlite, L. , and Gullion, D.  Cancer Res. (1974) 34, 1982-1988.
83. Abelson, H. T. , Karlan, D. , and Penman, S.  Biochim. Biophys. Acta (1974) 349, 389-401.
84. Abakumova, O. Y. , Ugarova, T. Y. , Gorbacheva, L. B. , Kucenco, N. G. , Pilipenco, N. N. , Sokolova, I. S. , and Lerman, M. I.  Cancer Res. (1974) 34, 1542-1547.
85. Kleihues, P. , and Magee, P. N.  Biochem. J. (1973) 136, 303-309.
86. Hradec, J. , and Kolar, G. F.  Chem. -Biol. Interact. (1974) 8, 243-251.

87. Wheeler, G. P. , and Alexander, J. A. Cancer Res. (1974) **34**, 1957-1964.
88. Rosenoff, S. H. , Bostick, F. W. , DeVita, V. T. , and Young, R. C. Proc. Am. Assoc. Cancer Res. (1973) **14**, 77.
89. Young, R. C. Cell Tissue Kinet. (1973) **6**, 35-43.
90. Brereton, H. D. , Bryant, T. L. , and Young, R, C. Cancer Res. (1975) **35**, 2420-2425.
91. Lerman, M. I. , Abakumova, O. Yu. , Kucenco, N. G. , Gorbacheva, L. B. , Kukushkina, G. V. , and Serebryanyi, A. M. Cancer Res. (1974) **34**, 1536-1541.
92. Bhuyan, B. K. Cancer Res. (1970) **30**, 2017-2023.
93. Druckrey, H. , Schagen, B. , and Ivankovic, S. Z. Krebsforsch. (1970) **74**, 141-161.
94. Verly, W. G. Biochem. Pharmacol. (1974) **23**, 3-8.
95. Lawley, P. D. , Lethbridge, J. H. , Edwards, P. A. , and Shooter, K. V. J. Mol. Biol. (1969) **39**, 181-198.
96. Lawley, P. D. , and Brookes, P. Biochem. J. (1963) **89**, 127-138.
97. Verly, W. G. , Barbason, H. , Dusart, J. , and Petitpas-Dewandre, A. Biochim. Biophys. Acta (1967) **145**, 752-762.
98. Shooter, K. V. , Howse, R. , and Merrifield, R. K. Biochem. J. (1974) **137**, 313-317.
99. Tobey, R. A. , and Crissman, H. A. Cancer Res. (1975) **35**, 460-470.
100. Tobey, R. A. , Oka, M. S. , and Crissman, H. A. Eur. J. Cancer (1975) **11**, 433-441.
101. Tobey, R. A. Nature (1975) **254**, 245-247.
102. Barranco, S. C. , Novak, J. K. , and Humphrey, R. M. Cancer Res. (1973) **33**, 691-694.
103. Barranco, S. C. , Novak, J. K. , and Humphrey, R. M. Cancer Res. (1975) **35**, 1194-1204.
104. Hahn, G. M. , Gordon, L. F. , and Kurkjian, S. D. Cancer Res. (1974) **34**, 2373-2377.
105. Frei, J. V. , and Oliver, J. Exp. Cell Res. (1972) **70**, 49-56.
106. Bruce, W. R. , and Valeriote, F. A. "The Proliferation and Spread of Neoplastic Cells, " pp 409-420. The Williams and Wilkins Company, Baltimore, 1968.
107. van Putten, L. M. , Lelieveld, P. , and Kram-Idsenga, L. K. J. Cancer Chemother. Rept. Part 1 (1972) **56**, 691-700.
108. Wilkoff, L. J. , Dulmadge, E. A. , and Lloyd, H. H. J. Natl. Cancer Inst. (1972) **48**, 685-695.
109. Wilkoff, L. J. , Dixon, G. J. , Dulmadge, E. A. , and Schabel, F. M. , Jr. Cancer Chemother. Rept. Part 1 (1967) **51**, 7-18.

110. Kelly, F. , and Legator, M. Mutat. Res. (1971) **12**, 183-190.

111. Bhuyan, B. K. , Scheidt, L. G. , and Fraser, T. J. Cancer Res. (1972) **32**, 398-407.

112. Barranco, S. C. , and Humphrey, R. M. Cancer Res. (1971) **31**, 191-195.

113. Drewinko, B. , Brown, B. W. , and Gottlieb, J. A. Cancer Res. (1973) **33**, 2732-2736.

114. Rakieten, N. , Rakieten, M. L. , and Nadkarni, M. V. Cancer Chemother. Rept. Part 1 (1963) **29**, 91-98.

115. Rudas, B. Arzneim. -Forsch. (1972) **22**, 830-861.

116. Schein, P. , McMenamin, M. , and Anderson, T. Int. Cancer Congr. Abs. 11th 1974 (No. 3) 437-438.

117. Schein, P. S. Cancer Res. (1969) **29**, 1226-1232.

118. Bannister, B. J. Antibiot. (1972) **25**, 377-386.

119. Schein, P. S. , Cooney, D. A. , McMenamin, M. G. , and Anderson, T. Biochem. Pharmacol. (1973) **22**, 2625-2631.

120. Hinz, M. , Katsilambros, N. , Maier, V. , Schatz, H. , and Pfeiffer, E. F. FEBS Lett. (1973) **30**, 225-228.

121. Gunnarsson, R. , Berne, C. , and Hellerström, C. Biochem. J. (1974) **140**, 487-494.

121. Schein, P. S. , Cooney, D. A. , and Vernon, M. L. Cancer Res. (1967) **27**, 2324-2332.

123. Wheeler, G. P. , Bowdon, B. J. , and Hammack, W. J. Biochem. Biophys. Res. Commun. (1973) **54**, 1024-1029.

# INDEX

# INDEX